Challenging Cases in

Pediatric Emergency Medicine

John T. Kanegaye, MD, FAAP, FACEP

Loren G. Yamamoto, MD, MPH, MBA, FAAP, FACEP

American Academy of Pediatrics
141 Northwest Point Blvd
Elk Grove Village, IL 60007-1098

American Academy of Pediatrics Department of Marketing and Publications

Maureen DeRosa, MPA, Director, Department of Marketing and Publications

Mark Grimes, Director, Division of Product Development

Martha Cook, Senior Product Development Editor

Eileen Glasstetter, Manager, Product Development

Sandi King, MS, Director, Division of Publishing and Production Services

Shannan Martin, Print Production Specialist

Linda Diamond, Manager, Art Direction and Production

Jason Crase, Editorial Specialist

Jill Ferguson, Director, Division of Marketing

Linda Smessaert, Manager, Clinical and Professional Publications Marketing

Robert Herling, Director, Division of Sales

Library of Congress Control Number 2008941467
ISBN 978-1-58110-300-7
MA0444

The recommendations in this publication do not indicate an exclusive course of treatment or serve as a standard of medical care. Variations, taking into account individual circumstances, may be appropriate.

Brand names are furnished for identifying purposes only. No endorsement of the manufacturers or products listed is implied.

The authors have no financial relationship with Masimo.

Printed in China
9-228/rep1014

2 3 4 5 6 7 8 9 10

Table of Contents

Acknowledgments

The authors would like to thank the American Academy of Pediatrics (AAP) for its initiative in bringing interesting and instructive case presentations to its members. As authors, clinicians, and educators, we are fortunate to have been given the opportunity to share these instructive cases that are based on our personal experiences. As implied by the title of *Challenging Cases,* the cases represent uncommon conditions or less common presentations of common conditions. In assembling these cases, we have sought to provoke the reader to consider a broader set of diagnoses. However, we have framed our discussions with the intent of reinforcing an approach to pediatric emergency medicine in which recognition and stabilization of the most dangerous conditions can occur simultaneously with evaluation and treatment of the most likely and the most important diagnoses suggested by a patient's presentation. We hope that practitioners and their patients will benefit from these case presentations and discussions. While we have tried to describe practices that are consistent with AAP policies and current evidence, such policies and medical knowledge change periodically and we are unable to review all such materials personally. A particular thanks to our technical reviewer, Ian McCaslin, MD, whose insights and suggestions strengthened the book considerably. Through the extraordinary efforts of AAP staff members Martha Cook, Eileen Glasstetter, and other editorial and publications staff, this has been an efficient and productive experience that demonstrates the dedication of the AAP to improving the quality of care provided to children.

John T. Kanegaye, MD, FAAP, FACEP
Loren G. Yamamoto, MD, MPH, MBA, FAAP, FACEP

Part 1

Gastrointestinal or Abdominal Presentations

Chapter 1

Projectile Vomiting in a 3-week-old

Presentation

A 3-week-old boy is brought to the emergency department because he has been vomiting for 3 days without improvement. The vomiting is characterized as "projectile" by his mother, and it is nonbilious. He feeds about 2 ounces (60 mL) per feeding. No fever or diarrhea is present.

Past medical, social, and family histories are not contributory.

Examination of vital signs reveals the following: rectal temperature 37.8°C, pulse 140 beats/min, respiration 35 breaths/min, blood pressure 60/40 mm Hg, and oxygen saturation 99% in room air. He weighs 3.2 kg. He is not as chubby as most infants. No distress is evident. Examination of head, eyes, ears, nose, and throat reveals slightly sticky oral mucosa and eyes that appear slightly sunken. Anterior fontanelle is soft but not sunken. His neck is supple, his heartbeat is regular, and his lungs are clear. His abdomen is soft and flat, with normal bowel sounds. There is a questionable olive-shaped mass that is palpated during feeding. He moves all his extremities well, and his tone is good. Color and perfusion are also good.

Discussion

Differential Diagnosis
- Pyloric stenosis
- Adrenal crisis (congenital adrenal hyperplasia)
- Bowel obstruction
- Meningitis
- Urinary tract infection
- Gastroenteritis

Evaluation
An initial abdominal radiograph series shows no evidence of obstruction. The stomach is not obviously dilated. Abdominal ultrasonography is negative for pyloric stenosis.

Laboratory evaluation is performed. His complete blood count is normal. Chemistry results show the following findings: glucose 50 mg/dL, sodium 131 mmol/L, potassium 6.1 mmol/L, chloride 98 mmol/L, bicarbonate 14 mmol/L, urinalysis specific gravity 1.030, moderate ketones, 0 to 1 white blood cells per high-power field.

Treatment
An intravenous (IV) line is started. The patient is given a rapid IV fluid infusion of normal saline and his glucose is corrected. He is given IV methylprednisolone and oral fludrocortisone.

The final diagnosis is adrenal crisis, congenital adrenal hyperplasia, and 21-hydroxylase deficiency.

Keep in Mind
Although the clinical manifestation is suggestive of pyloric stenosis, the patient's imaging studies are not consistent with pyloric stenosis. Are the results of the laboratory studies consistent with pyloric stenosis?

Most patients with pyloric stenosis have hyponatremia, hypokalemia, and a metabolic alkalosis. If the degree of dehydration is more severe, a metabolic acidosis will develop. However, in this case, there is hypoglycemia, hyponatremia, and hyperkalemia. All of these findings are consistent with a salt-losing adrenal crisis (addisonian crisis).

Asking parents whether the vomiting is projectile in nature can be misleading because all vomiting projects. It is more specific to ask whether the vomit can hit the wall if standing 1 m from it. Nonprojectile vomiting does not hit the wall, whereas truly projectile vomiting does.

An adrenal crisis is an acute deficiency of corticosteroids (glucocorticoids) and mineralocorticoids. Glucocorticoid deficiency results in feeling acutely ill and vomiting, hypoglycemia, and further deterioration resembling acute shock. Mineralocorticoid deficiency results in hyponatremia and hyperkalemia. The hyperkalemia can be high enough to result in an acute nonperfusing dysrhythmia.

Severe hyperkalemia is an emergency. A nonperfusing rhythm can be reversed with IV calcium. This will restore a perfusing rhythm temporarily, but the serum potassium level must be reduced before the effect of the IV calcium wears off. The usually recommended therapies to rapidly reduce potassium levels are IV sodium bicarbonate, albuterol aerosol, and IV insulin. All of these work by redistributing potassium from the extracellular space to the intracellular space. Sodium bicarbonate reduces the level of acidosis. Alkalosis drives potassium intracellularly. Acidosis drives potassium extracellularly. Albuterol is an adrenergic that can be administered safely, and this also drives potassium intracellularly. Insulin drives potassium intracellularly, but this will result in hypoglycemia, so a glucose infusion must be administered concurrently with frequent bedside glucose measurements. Of these treatments, the 2 that can be delivered immediately (because of immediate availability) are IV sodium bicarbonate and albuterol aerosol. Once these measures are in place, removing potassium from the body with furosemide and sodium-potassium exchange resin can be initiated.

The acute glucocorticoid deficiency can be treated with a standard pharmacologic loading dose of corticosteroids such as IV methylprednisolone. The acute mineralocorticoid deficiency can be treated with a pharmacologic mineralocorticoid. Although IV hydrocortisone has some mineralocorticoid activity, it might not be sufficient. Fludrocortisone can be given for higher potency and long-term mineralocorticoid activity.

Most patients with congenital adrenal hyperplasia in an acute adrenal crisis have 21-hydroxylase deficiency. The metabolic pathways lead to high levels of androgenic steroids. Female patients with 21-hydroxylase deficiency are born with virilized (ie, masculinized) external genitalia or ambiguous genitalia. This finding prompts medical attention, and the diagnosis of congenital adrenal hyperplasia in girls is generally identified in the newborn nursery. Boys have normal-appearing genitalia, and thus congenital adrenal hyperplasia is generally not evident until they experience an acute adrenal crisis.

The long-term management of these patients in balancing their glucocorticoid and mineralocorticoid doses is a difficult task. The emergency department management focuses on establishing the diagnosis, treating the glucocorticoid and mineralocorticoid deficiencies, correcting hypoglycemia and dehydration, and preventing complications from severe hyperkalemia.

Recommended Reading

Agus MS. Endocrine emergencies. In: Fleisher GR, Ludwig S, Henretig FM, Ruddy RM, Silverman BK, eds. *Textbook of Pediatric Emergency Medicine.* 5th ed. Philadelphia, PA: Lippincott Williams & Wilkins; 2006:1167–1192

Glaser N, Enns GM, Kupperman N. Metabolic disease. In: Gausche-Hill M, Fuchs S, Yamamoto L, eds. *APLS: The Pediatric Emergency Medicine Resource.* 4th rev ed. Sudbury, MA: Jones and Bartlett Publishers; 2007:186–207

Chapter 2

Vomiting in a 1-month-old

Presentation

A 1-month-old boy is brought to the emergency department because he has experienced 5 vomiting episodes today. His appetite is decreased. He is fussy and difficult to console. There is no history of fever, diarrhea, or contact with people who are ill.

A third-year medical student is sent to examine the patient, and he reports the following findings: past medical, social, and family histories are not contributory. Examination reveals the following vital signs: rectal temperature 38.6°C, pulse 140 beats/min, and respiration 40 breaths/min. The baby is crying, fussy, and difficult to console, but he is well developed and nourished. His oral mucosa is moist. His neck is supple, his heartbeat is regular, and his lungs are clear. His abdomen is soft and flat, with normal bowel sounds. He moves all his extremities, and his facial function is good.

Discussion

Differential Diagnosis
- Viral infection
- Meningitis
- Bowel obstruction
- Pyloric stenosis
- Adrenal crisis
- Sepsis

Evaluation
Laboratory evaluation is performed, with the following findings: sodium 131 mmol/L, potassium 3.2 mmol/L, chloride 94 mmol/L, bicarbonate 23 mmol/L, glucose 79 mg/dL, urinalysis specific gravity 1.024, small ketones, and 0 to 1 white blood cells per high-power field. Complete blood count revealed white blood cells 13,500/μL, with 35% segmented neutrophils, 2% bands, 50% lymphocytes, 13% monocytes, hemoglobin 14 g/dL, hematocrit 48%, and an increased platelet count. Lumbar puncture is performed, and analysis of cerebrospinal fluid is normal. An abdominal series is ordered. Cultures of blood, urine, and cerebrospinal fluid are obtained, and intravenous antibiotics administered.

Figure 2-1 shows findings typical of a bowel obstruction. The black arrow points to an area that looks like a gas pocket trapped in the patient's left groin. This is probably some type of artifact, but it prompts the attending physician to open the patient's diaper, where an incarcerated inguinal hernia is in plain view.

Treatment
The inguinal hernia cannot be reduced. A consulted pediatric surgeon is not able to reduce the inguinal hernia. The patient undergoes an inguinal hernia reduction and repair. He subsequently does well.

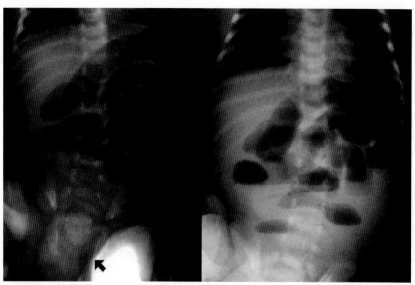

Figure 2-1

Keep in Mind

Incarcerated inguinal hernias are known causes of vomiting and represent a surgical emergency. All patients with a history of vomiting should be examined in their groin and genital region to confirm the absence of an incarcerated inguinal hernia.

Four radiographic criteria for identifying a bowel obstruction are bowel gas distribution, bowel distention, air fluid levels, and orderliness. In this particular patient, the bowel gas distribution is present in all areas of the abdomen. The bowel is clearly distended, as evidenced by the smooth bowel walls. The bowel resembles large sausages or hoses. Distention is not assessed by measuring the bowel diameter but rather by recognizing the loss of bowel haustration and plication, resulting in a smooth, sausage-like bowel. The air fluid levels are best assessed on the upright view (Figure 2-1 right). Air fluid levels are clearly present. Two air fluid levels within the same loop of bowel are known as a J-turn, a hairpin loop, or a candy cane, and are highly indicative of a bowel obstruction. Orderliness refers to the randomness of gas distribution. Most infant abdominal radiographs have lots of gas that resembles popcorn because the bowel plications and haustrations are preserved. This disorderliness is less likely to be present in a bowel obstruction. However, orderliness resembles a bag of sausages, and this finding is more likely to be present in a bowel obstruction. A simpler way to assess this is, does the gas pattern resemble a bag of popcorn or a bag of sausages? This clearly looks like a bag of sausages. Three out of the 4 criteria, therefore, strongly point to a bowel obstruction.

The causes of a bowel obstruction can be remembered with the mnemonic AIM (or more accurately, AAIIMM): adhesions, appendicitis, intussusception, incarcerated inguinal hernia, Meckel diverticulum, and malrotation (with midgut volvulus).

Recommended Reading

Chan-Nishina CC, Tim-Sing PML. Test your skill in distinguishing obstruction from ileus. In: Yamamoto LG, Inaba AS, DiMauro R, eds. *Radiology Cases in Pediatric Emergency Medicine.* Vol 3, case 18. August 1995. Available at: http://www.hawaii.edu/medicine/pediatrics/pemxray/v3c18.html. Accessed December 9, 2008

Yamamoto LG. Failure to thrive and vomiting in a 1-month-old. In: Yamamoto LG, Inaba AS, DiMauro R, eds. *Radiology Cases in Pediatric Emergency Medicine.* Vol 3, case 16. August 1995. Available at: http://www.hawaii.edu/medicine/pediatrics/pemxray/v3c16.html. Accessed December 9, 2008

Chapter 3

Vomiting Following Intussusception Reduction

Presentation

A 5-month-old girl seeks care at a rural emergency department (ED) with vomiting and colicky abdominal pain. A barium enema confirmed an ileocolic intussusception, which was successfully reduced by the radiologist who performed the barium enema. Her symptoms have largely resolved. The rural ED is now calling to transfer the patient to a children's hospital for evaluation by a pediatric surgeon and overnight hospitalization. The children's hospital accepts the patient transfer, although it seems likely that this patient should do well if the intussusception has been successfully reduced.

She arrives in the middle of the night, and her examination, which is performed by house staff, is unremarkable. The pediatric surgeon is called.

Later that morning, the pediatric surgeon evaluates the patient and finds the patient to be doing well. She no longer needs to be kept fasting and she seems hungry, so she is started on clear fluids and then formula feeding. She is about to be discharged from the hospital when she vomits once. Her examination continues to be benign.

Discussion

Differential Diagnosis
- Recurrence of intussusception
- Gastroenteritis
- Overfeeding

Evaluation
An abdominal series is ordered (Figure 3-1).

There is some residual barium from the previous evening's barium enema. The gas distribution is not reassuring. The surgeon orders an ultrasound, but before this study can be done, the child is noted to be feeding well and no further vomiting has occurred. Observation is continued, and she does well. She is discharged in the evening.

The next morning, the radiologist reviews all the radiographs from the weekend and calls to notify the surgeon of an important radiographic finding. The patient is noted to have a dislocated left hip (Figure 3-2). In young infants, the femur head has not ossified, making the identification of a hip dislocation difficult. Several diagrammatic schemes have been devised to

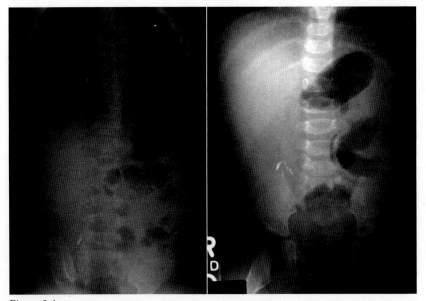

Figure 3-1

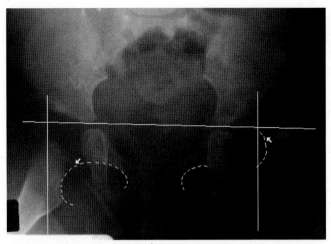

Figure 3-2

identify dislocations. The easiest of these is to identify the Shenton arc. The arc is drawn as an oval from the obturator foramen (medial portion of the arc) to the medial portion of the proximal femur. The Shenton arc in the patient's right hip is contiguous, but the Shenton arc in the patient's left hip is clearly not contiguous, indicating that the left hip is dislocated.

Treatment
The patient is referred to an orthopedic surgeon for management of the congenital dislocated hip.

Keep in Mind
Congenital hip dislocation is part of the spectrum of congenital dysplasia of the hip. Hip dysplasia can range from a barely detectable instability of the hip to a nonreducible dislocation of the hip. Very mild cases may resolve on their own without any long-term morbidity. More severe cases result in the progression of symptoms and if not diagnosed at an early stage, can lead to an irreversibly damaged hip.

Early diagnosis and treatment of congenital hip dysplasia are required to prevent permanent injury to the hip. Physicians providing primary care for infants routinely screen for hip dysplasia. However, there is no clinical finding or screening method that can reliably detect all cases. For this reason, patients with hip dysplasia might be discovered during assessments for abdominal conditions not related to hip dysplasia. If an abdominal radiograph is ordered on such a patient, the diagnosis may be apparent radiographically if one is astute enough to survey the bony structures.

Failing to identify a congenital hip dislocation on a radiograph may result in liability if the patient's condition is ultimately diagnosed after the patient experiences irreversible hip damage. Protection from liability is not necessarily afforded, even if the radiograph was ordered for a different reason.

Most infants with congenital hip dysplasia can be detected by routine screening. This responsibility rests largely with primary care physicians. However, not all children have access to a primary care physician. Infant growth and development change the musculoskeletal structure of the hip such that screening examination measures become less reliable in detecting hip dysplasia as the infant grows. The Ortolani and Barlow signs have usually disappeared by 6 weeks of age. Detection of congenital hip dysplasia outside of this age relies on the identification of subtle findings such as lower extremity length asymmetry; loss of the normal hip flexion contracture; buttock fullness; a hollow anterior groin; asymmetry of the perineal, gluteal, or thigh folds and creases; or a palpably dislocated femoral head.

Recommended Reading

American Academy of Pediatrics Committee on Quality Improvement, Subcommittee on Developmental Dysplasia of the Hip. Clinical practice guideline: early detection of developmental dysplasia of the hip. *Pediatrics.* 2000;105:896–905

Durkin RC. Hip conditions. In: Yamamoto LG, Inaba AS, Okamoto JK, Patronis ME, Yamashiroya VK, eds. *Case Based Pediatrics for Medical Students and Residents.* Honolulu, HI: University of Hawaii; 2004:601–605. Available at: http://www.hawaii.edu/medicine/pediatrics/pedtext. Accessed December 10, 2008

Yamamoto LG. Vomiting following reduction of intussusception. In: Yamamoto LG, Inaba AS, DiMauro R, eds. *Radiology Cases in Pediatric Emergency Medicine.* Vol 2, case 13. March 1995. Available at: http://www.hawaii.edu/medicine/pediatrics/pemxray/v2c13.html. Accessed December 10, 2008

Chapter 4

Vomiting and Diarrhea 1

Presentation

A 2-year-old girl is brought to the emergency department (ED) by her mother because of vomiting and diarrhea. She has vomited 15 times in the past 10 hours. She is less active, and her mother thinks that she last urinated 7 hours ago, although she is not sure because of the diarrhea. No fever has been noted. The mother has been giving her apple juice, but she vomits it up most of the time, and at other times, she refuses to drink.

Past medical history is negative. Family history is significant because of an older brother who had some vomiting and diarrhea 4 days ago, but his symptoms were not as bad, and he has since recovered.

Examination reveals the following vital signs: rectal temperature 37.8°C, pulse 145 beats/min, respiration 24 breaths/min, blood pressure 90/40 mm Hg, and oxygen saturation 99% in room air. The patient is drowsy and subdued, but she wakes up when examined. Her oral mucosa is sticky. Tympanic membranes are normal. Her neck is supple. Her heartbeat is regular with no murmur. Her lungs are clear. Her abdomen is soft and flat with normal bowel sounds. There are no inguinal hernias. Her external genitalia are normal. Perfusion is good. Capillary refill time is 1.5 to 2 seconds. She is moving all extremities well with good muscle tone.

Discussion

Differential Diagnosis
- Gastroenteritis
- Oliguria
- Dehydration
- Bowel obstruction

Evaluation
Some evaluation and treatment issues to decide on include the following:

- How dehydrated is this person and does this affect the therapeutic decisions?
- Should this patient be given intravenous (IV) fluids or oral rehydration?
- How much fluid is necessary to rehydrate her and how fast should this be given?
- Is there a role for antiemetics such as ondansetron?
- Is there a role for antidiarrheal agents such as loperamide?

The patient is assessed as having mild dehydration most likely caused by viral gastroenteritis. She is a good candidate for oral rehydration and oral hydration maintenance.

Treatment
She is given oral ondansetron. Twenty minutes later, she is given a flavored electrolyte solution, which she drinks eagerly, although she is limited to 30 to 40 mL at a time every 10 to 15 minutes. She is also given crackers. She continues to do well over the next 45 minutes, at which point her parents request that she be discharged from the ED. They will continue the fluids and feedings at home and return if her condition worsens.

Keep in Mind

This patient appears to be mildly dehydrated. Most textbooks describe dehydration severity by symptoms. Patients with 5% dehydration usually have no tears when crying, oliguria, sticky oral mucosa, and less energy and activity levels. Patients with 10% dehydration have sunken eyes and diminished skin turgor. Patients with 15% dehydration have signs including

obvious shock (eg, tachycardia, hypotension, cool extremities) and tenting
of the skin. However, it is difficult to confirm the accuracy of dehydration
levels in children because baseline weights are nearly impossible to obtain
as a result of varying degrees of growth and lean body mass weight loss
during the illness and convalescence.

If this patient is classified as having a more severe level of dehydration,
a common recommendation is to administer IV fluid rehydration. This
provides certainty that the patient's hydration status will improve (at least
temporarily), reducing or eliminating the risk of complications from
worsening dehydration.

Patients with mild dehydration can usually be offered a choice of IV versus
oral hydration. An adult feeling miserable and nauseated might prefer to
lie down and relax while receiving IV fluids as opposed to drinking salty
electrolyte solutions. Contrast this with a young child, who might prefer
oral fluids to an IV needle in the arm.

If IV fluid therapy is chosen, normal saline or lactated Ringer solution
should be infused. A general approach is to start with 20 mL/kg, which
replaces 2% of the body weight (20 mL/kg = 20 mL/1,000 g, which is
approximately 20 mL per 1,000 mL, which = 2 mL/100 mL = 2%). If this
patient is 4% dehydrated, she will need 40 mL/kg to be fully hydrated; the
40 mL/kg does not, however, address her 24-hour maintenance fluid needs
(100 mL/kg for the first 10 kg; 50 mL/kg for the next 10 kg; 20 mL/kg
thereafter), so she probably will need more than 40 mL/kg.

It is prudent to start with 40 mL/kg infused over 1 to 2 hours as a minimum
if an IV is placed, because 20 mL/kg is a small volume of fluid. If the patient
weighs 15 kg, her IV rate is 300 mL/h for 2 hours (total 600 mL = 40 mL/kg
total). Alternatively, she could receive 600 mL/h for 1 hour. The lower IV
rate is preferred by some because it gives caregivers time to determine
whether her overall status is improving or worsening. In crowded ED facilities, a faster infusion rate makes sense. In ED facilities that can afford additional observation time, a 2-hour infusion has an observational advantage.
Although these IV rates sound fast, they are only 20 mL/kg per hour to
40 mL/kg per hour, which replace 2% to 4% of the body weight per hour.
This can more easily be appreciated if translated to soda-can equivalents.

A typical soda can is 12 ounces (360 mL). Three hundred mL per hour is less than one soda can per hour, which does not seem to be very fast. An IV should not be started unless the plan is to administer at least 40 mL/kg (4% of the body weight fluid replacement). Less than this volume can more easily be accomplished via the oral route in most instances. In other words, in this 2-year-old, an IV should not be started if the plan is to administer a mere one soda can's volume of fluid. That is a waste of IV equipment charges and subjects the patient to the pain and discomfort of an IV to administer the volume of a soda can.

Ondansetron can play a minor to substantial therapeutic role. Oral and IV ondansetron work well. It can also be administered intramuscularly (IM), but this is usually not necessary. Patients with a history of migraine headaches or children with a family history of migraine headaches should be cautioned about the possibility that ondansetron could precipitate a headache. A common protocol is to administer ondansetron (0.15 mg/kg orally up to 4 mg, although 8 mg is given to some adults), then 20 minutes later start a trial of oral fluids to see whether the patient improves. In most instances, patients are less nauseated and will not vomit if they drink small amounts at a time. If the patient vomits up the oral ondansetron, it can be readministered orally or IM.

Ondansetron is available in a dissolvable pill, called an oral disintegrating tablet (ODT). The smallest ODT is 4 mg, so it is not too hard to give 2 mg (half of an ODT tablet), but smaller doses should probably be provided using the liquid preparation. Oral ondansetron can be tried in the out-patient clinic or office for willing patients as an option before referring the patient to an ED.

The American Academy of Pediatrics does not support the use of anti-diarrheal agents such as loperamide.

Recommended Reading

Freedman SB, Adler M, Seshadri R, Powell EC. Oral ondansetron for gastroenteritis in a pediatric emergency department. *N Engl J Med.* 2006;354:1698–1705

King CK, Glass R, Bresee JS, Duggan C; Centers for Disease Control and Prevention. Managing acute gastroenteritis among children: oral rehydration, maintenance, and nutritional therapy. *MMWR Recomm Rep.* 2003;52(RR-16):1–16. Available at: http://www.cdc.gov/mmwr/preview/ mmwrhtml/rr5216a1.htm. Accessed December 10, 2008. AAP endorsed

Ramsook C, Sahagun-Carreon I, Kozinetz CA, Moro-Sutherland D. A randomized clinical trial comparing oral ondansetron with placebo in children with vomiting from acute gastroenteritis. *Ann Emerg Med.* 2002;39:397–403

Yamamoto LG. Fluids and electrolytes. In: Yamamoto LG, Inaba AS, Okamoto JK, Patronis ME, Yamashiroya VK, eds. *Case Based Pediatrics for Medical Students and Residents.* Honolulu, HI: University of Hawaii; 2004:46–51. Available at: http://www.hawaii.edu/medicine/pediatrics/ pedtext. Accessed December 10, 2008

Chapter 5

Vomiting and Diarrhea 2

Presentation

A 2-year-old girl is brought to the emergency department (ED) by her
mother because of vomiting and diarrhea. She has vomited 10 times in
the past 7 hours. She is less active than usual. Her mother thinks that she
last urinated 5 hours ago, although she is not sure because of the diarrhea
(5 episodes, nonbloody). No fever has been noted. Her parents have tried
oral fluid hydration on the advice of a telephone recommendation from
her primary care practitioner, but she not been able to hold down even
small volumes of fluid.

Past medical history is significant for anemia. She is supposed to be taking
multiple vitamin drops containing iron and fluoride, but the drops ran out
one month ago and the prescription has not been refilled. No history of
urinary infections is present.

Examination reveals the following vital signs: rectal temperature 37.8°C,
pulse 185 beats/min, and respiration 46 breaths/min (while crying). Blood
pressure is not obtainable because of crying. Oxygen saturation is 99% in
room air. She is awake and cooperative but drowsy and subdued. Mild
pallor is noted. Her oral mucosa is moist, but she vomited 15 minutes ago.
Tympanic membranes are slightly red. Her neck is supple. Her heart is
tachycardic with no obvious murmur. Her lungs are clear. Her abdomen
is soft and flat with normal bowel sounds. It is difficult to feel a liver edge.
There are no inguinal hernias. Perfusion is good. Capillary refill time is
1.5 to 2 seconds. She is moving all extremities well with good muscle tone.

Discussion

Differential Diagnosis

- Gastroenteritis, probably viral
- Oliguria due to dehydration
- Anemia

Evaluation

Intravenous (IV) fluid hydration versus oral fluid hydration options are discussed with the patient's parents. Because her parents have not been able to get her to hold down even small volumes of fluid, they request that IV fluid hydration in the ED be initiated.

Laboratory analysis reveals the following: sodium 135 mmol/L, potassium 5.0 mmol/L, chloride 99 mmol/L, bicarbonate 19 mmol/L, and glucose 130 mg/dL. Complete blood count (CBC) is performed, with the following findings: white blood cells 12,000/μL, 60% segmented neutrophils, 5% bands, 25% lymphocytes, 10% monocytes, hemoglobin 9 g/dL, hematocrit 27%, and platelets 140,000/μL.

Treatment

Intravenous normal saline is infused at 20 mL/kg per hour for 2 hours. After hydration, the patient is no longer vomiting. She still looks pale. She has not voided, so the IV fluids are continued. She is fussy and cries intermittently. Her eyes are moist and she has tears. Her eyes look slightly puffy, but this is attributed to the crying.

You think that some clinical parameters are not consistent with gastroenteritis and mild dehydration. Although she is crying with lots of tears and her eyes appear to be puffy, she has still not voided. Additionally, the pallor appears to be excessive for someone with a hemoglobin of 9 g/dL. Mild dehydration and mild anemia could cause a patient to look visibly pale, but although her hydration status should be improving, her pallor has not gotten better. You decide to repeat her CBC and check her renal function because she has still not voided.

The follow-up CBC has the following results: white blood cells 13,000/μL, 70% segmented neutrophils, 4% bands, 15% lymphocytes, 11% monocytes, hemoglobin 6.5 g/dL, hematocrit 19.5%, and platelet count 90,000/μL. Blood urea nitrogen is 55 mg/dL and creatinine 4.5 mg/dL.

Her hemoglobin and platelet count are declining further. Significant azotemia (not simply prerenal) is present. Her IV fluid volume infusion is reduced, and she is hospitalized in the intensive care unit for further management.

You diagnose her with hemolytic uremic syndrome (HUS).

Keep in Mind

Hemolytic uremic syndrome is characterized by a combination of micro-angiopathic hemolytic anemia, variable degrees of thrombocytopenia, and renal failure. Other organ systems can be affected as well. Diarrhea-associated HUS and atypical nondiarrheal HUS appear to be different entities, with the latter having a worse prognosis. It is likely that HUS consists of a heterogenous group of disorders that have similar characteristics.

Shigella gastroenteritis and *Escherichia coli* O157 have the greatest known link to HUS. *E coli* O157 usually presents with bloody diarrhea. A common source of *E coli* O157 is animal fecal contamination. Outbreaks in the United States have been caused by contaminated ground beef that was not fully cooked, contaminated vegetables, and contaminated fruit juice that was not pasteurized.

Patients with *E coli* O157 or other causes of gastroenteritis do not necessarily have HUS when they initially seek care. Hemolytic uremic syndrome can develop 1 to 15 days later.

The treatment for HUS is largely supportive. Before the availability of dialysis, many patients died from renal failure. Dialysis improves complications as a result of renal dysfunction. Most children with HUS will recover completely. Varying degrees of chronic renal disease will persist in some patients.

Thrombotic thrombocytopenic purpura is similar to HUS; both have the same clinical triad. Thrombotic thrombocytopenic purpura is more serious and affects more organ systems. Thrombotic thrombocytopenic purpura and HUS are likely to have some common pathophysiological processes.

Recommended Reading

Cronan KM, Kost SI. Renal and electrolyte emergencies. In: Fleisher GR, Ludwig S, Henretig FM, Ruddy RM, Silverman BK, eds. *Textbook of Pediatric Emergency Medicine*. 5th ed. Philadelphia, PA: Lippincott Williams & Wilkins, 2006:873–919

Marr JK. Hemolytic uremic syndrome. In: Yamamoto LG, Inaba AS, Okamoto JK, Patronis ME, Yamashiroya VK, eds. *Case Based Pediatrics for Medical Students and Residents*. Honolulu, HI: University of Hawaii; 2004:433–435. Available at: http://www.hawaii.edu/medicine/pediatrics/pedtext. Accessed December 10, 2008

Chapter 6

Vomiting and Dizziness After a Banquet

Presentation

Two families arrive in the emergency department (ED) simultaneously. They have both come from a wedding reception dinner. After dinner, they began feeling ill; eventually, all of them were in the bathroom of the banquet hall, vomiting. They began feeling weak and dizzy, so they drove to the hospital ED. They were all well before eating dinner. One family has 2 children; the other has 3. There are 9 patients total. They were all sitting at the same table at the wedding dinner.

Past medical histories are variable but largely negative.

Examination findings are also variable but include mild dehydration, discomfort, and nausea. Mild tachycardia and normal blood pressures are recorded. Strength testing is normal. Sensory testing reveals no deficits.

As you rush to complete these 9 charts, the triage nurse informs you that one more patient has come in with similar symptoms, and he was at the same wedding dinner. However, in this case, his parents and siblings are not ill.

Discussion

Differential Diagnosis
- Food poisoning

Evaluation
Food poisoning is the only reasonable diagnosis. It would be very difficult for any other process to result in such a rapid onset of symptoms in such a finite group in such close proximity.

The 10th patient provides a substantial clue to identifying the offending food agent. Because the first 9 patients were seated at the same table, they all ate the same food. Thus, it is not possible to determine which food it was. It is interesting that only one other patient at the banquet became ill. This suggests that it is not likely to have been a food preparation problem because large amounts of the prepared food would likely have been distributed to many others in the banquet hall. However, it is also possible that there are many other patients who have sought care in other EDs or who have gone home with milder symptoms and are not seeking emergency care. In addition to geographic proximity, specialty patient services (eg, a children's hospital) or health maintenance organization restrictions affect the selection of an emergency care facility.

The 9-course dinner menu served was a combination of American and Asian dishes consisting of clam chowder, Caesar salad, vegetables and shrimp, sliced sirloin steak, crab legs, steamed fish, roast pork, chow fun noodles, and dessert (cake and ice cream).

The 10th patient is a 12-year-old boy who is a cousin of the children in the other 2 families. He states that he moved to their table to eat with them for about 20 minutes. While he sat with them, he ate the fish and noodles.

At this point, ciguatera fish poisoning is suspected.

Treatment
Intravenous (IV) fluid infusions are started in all the patients. Antiemetic agents are administered to some patients, with variable degrees of improvement. However, improvement is also noted in patients who did not receive antiemetics.

Keep in Mind

Ciguatera toxin is produced by tiny marine organisms called dinoflagellates. Toxin production by these organisms seems to surge at varying times as a result of factors that are not well understood. Smaller fish consume the dinoflagellates. The toxin is not digested but rather stored in the flesh. The smaller fish are consumed by larger fish. Fish consuming large amounts of toxin store higher concentrations of the toxin in their flesh. The toxin is not harmful to the fish. Human ciguatera food poisoning occurs when the flesh from such fish is consumed. The ciguatera toxin is heat stable, so cooking the fish does not denature the toxin. Although steamed fish was served to all tables at the banquet, a single large fish was served at each table. It appears that only this particular fish contained enough ciguatera toxin to make these 2 families ill.

Although ciguatera is usually described as occurring in fish in the tropics or the southern United States, today these fish are shipped all over the world, making geographic epidemiology less applicable.

Ciguatera poisoning is uncommon. A cluster of cases often manifests (all those who ate the fish), prompting consideration of ciguatera as the cause. Symptoms can begin shortly after eating the fish or can be delayed by several hours. Initially, patients develop nausea, vomiting, diarrhea, and abdominal cramps. Neurologic symptoms will often follow later, including paresthesia, weakness, and altered sensorium. One of the symptoms that is classically attributed to ciguatera is reversal of hot-cold sensation, so hot items feel cold and vice versa. Most publications do not state how common this is.

Treatment is largely supportive. It's a good idea to hospitalize patients because the acute effects are likely to persist for a day or more, and many patients will go on to have prolonged paresthesia and neurologic symptoms. Intravenous mannitol may be used to treat the patients, although IV fluids alone may be sufficient. Gabapentin therapy may alleviate neurologic symptoms during convalescence.

Recommended Reading

Salerno DA, Aronoff SC. Nonbacterial food poisoning. In: Kliegman RM, Behrman RE, Jenson HB, Stanton BF, eds. *Nelson Textbook of Pediatrics.* 18th ed. Int ed. Philadelphia, PA: WB Saunders; 2007:2118–2921

Osterhoudt KC, Ewald MB, Shannon M, Henretig FM. Toxicologic emergencies. In: Fleisher GR, Ludwig S, Henretig FM, Ruddy RM, Silverman BK, eds. *Textbook of Pediatric Emergency Medicine.* 5th ed. Philadelphia, PA: Lippincott Williams & Wilkins; 2006:951–1007

Perez CM, Vasquez PA, Perret CF. Treatment of ciguatera poisoning with gabapentin. *N Engl J Med.* 2001;344:692–693

Schnorf H, Taurarii M, Cundy T. Ciguatera fish poisoning: a double-blind randomized trial of mannitol therapy. *Neurology.* 2002;58:873–880

Chapter 7

Premature Infant With Bloody Stools and Shock

Presentation

This 2-month-old infant, born at 28 weeks' gestational age, has had abdominal distention and 3 to 4 episodes of bloody stools over the last 6 hours. This patient was brought to another hospital passing bright red blood from his rectum. There, the infant was tachycardic and tachypneic, with signs of poor perfusion. An abdominal radiograph demonstrated distended bowel loops, resulting in transfer to your emergency department (ED) for further evaluation. Before transport, his hematocrit was 39%. During transport, the child received 40 mL/kg of normal saline. His systolic blood pressure remained normal (≥92 mm Hg), and heart rate was 142 to 154 beats/min through transport. The infant was recently discharged after a prolonged but uneventful neonatal intensive care course with no history of abdominal surgery or complications of prematurity.

On arrival at your ED, the patient is afebrile with a heart rate of 140 beats/min, respiratory rate of 80 breaths/min, blood pressure of 91/76 mm Hg, and room air oxyhemoglobin saturation of 98%. He is fussy and appears to be in distress, with grunting and retractions. The abdomen is tensely distended and tympanitic; bowel sounds are absent. Blood is present at the anus, but there is no evidence of trauma or fissure. Femoral and radial pulses are normal, but the skin is mottled and cool, with delayed capillary refill.

Discussion

Differential Diagnosis
- Necrotizing enterocolitis
- Intussusception
- Midgut volvulus
- Trauma
- Meckel diverticulum
- Infection
- Milk protein intolerance
- Hirschsprung disease
- Anal fissure
- Swallowed maternal blood
- Coagulopathy

Evaluation
Laboratory analysis reveals the following values: white blood cell count 12,500/μL, hemoglobin 10.6 g/dL, platelets 369,000/μL, venous pH 7.29, P_{CO_2} 46 mm Hg, and base excess -5 mmol/L. Repeat radiographs continue to show dilated loops but no mass, pneumatosis intestinalis, or free intraperitoneal air (Figure 7-1).

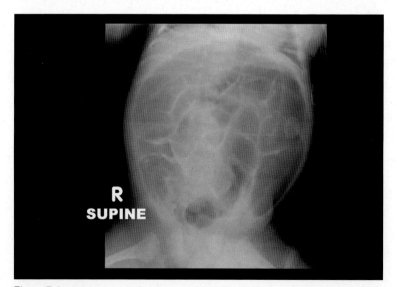

Figure 7-1

Treatment

Your patient is in compensated shock. You immediately provide additional fluid resuscitation, which results in an improvement in perfusion. You begin other supportive measures including warming lights and gastric decompression by nasogastric tube. The gastric aspirate is nonbloody. Because of the risk of bowel compromise, meropenem is administered. After stabilization in the ED, the patient is admitted to the pediatric intensive care unit where he is met by a surgical consultant. A contrast enema reveals an obstructing mass in the distal sigmoid colon, consistent with intussusception (Figure 7-2), that does not reduce beyond the proximal sigmoid colon. During a subsequent reduction attempt by air contrast

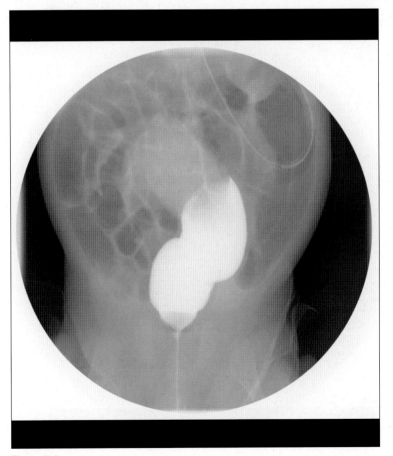

Figure 7-2

enema, a pneumoperitoneum develops (Figure 7-3) and the procedure is terminated. The patient undergoes open reduction of the intussusception with resection of a segment of perforated colon and creation of an ileostomy.

Keep in Mind

Many of the common causes of lower gastrointestinal bleeding in infancy are relatively benign (eg, anal fissure, milk protein intolerance, swallowed maternal blood). If the clinical examination is reassuring, then formal ED evaluation for less common but more worrisome causes becomes less urgent. Nonetheless, the clinician must carefully consider less common

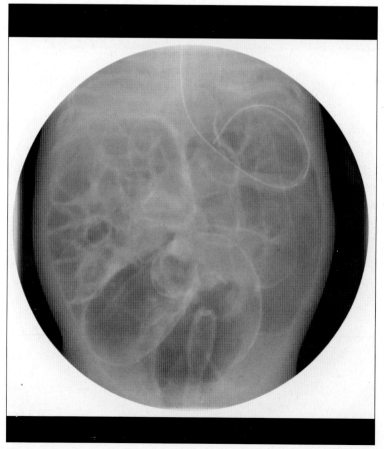

Figure 7-3

causes that require urgent intervention. When abnormalities are uncovered, the urgency for diagnostic evaluation, most typically in the form of radiologic studies, increases. When hemodynamic or respiratory compromise is present, resuscitation takes priority over diagnosis.

Although normotensive, this patient presents with clinical evidence of compensated shock. The pediatric patient has a tremendous capacity to sustain normal blood pressure until shock is far advanced. Tachycardia and vasoconstriction are the primary compensatory mechanisms and are more sensitive indicators of shock and response to therapy. Until the diagnosis of intussusception was known, the etiology could have included hypovolemia (due to hemorrhage or fluid shifts), sepsis, and impaired preload due to abdominal distension. Regardless of the etiology and specific physiologic disturbances leading to shock, support of hemodynamic status should be started without delay.

As in this case, rapid bolus infusion of isotonic fluid, repeated as guided by frequent reassessments, is appropriate initial therapy. Vasoactive infusions are appropriate if shock is refractory to volume resuscitation. If shock persists, particularly with evidence of respiratory compromise, mechanical ventilation is warranted. Warming measures are particularly important for small infants who are exposed for resuscitation and administered fluids that have not been warmed. Placement of a nasogastric tube will not only relieve abdominal distention, but also reduce the respiratory compromise and preload reduction that may occur as a result of displacement of abdominal contents. Examination of the aspirate helps to exclude an upper gastrointestinal source of bleeding.

The traditional diagnostic and therapeutic intervention for intussusception is the hydrostatic contrast enema. The classic barium enema is now often performed with water-soluble contrast. Air contrast, or pneumatic, reduction has gained popularity because of its perceived greater convenience, greater success rates, and decreased risk of intraperitoneal contamination in the event of perforation. However, when the initial diagnosis is uncertain or a pathologic lead point is likely, hydrostatic methods may have a greater diagnostic yield.

Recommended Reading

Arensman RM, Browne M, Madonna MB. Gastrointestinal bleeding. In: Grosfeld JL, O'Neill JA, Coran AG, Fonkalsrud EW, Caldamone AA, eds. *Pediatric Surgery.* 6th ed. Philadelphia, PA: Mosby Elsevier; 2006:1383–1388

Ein SH, Daneman A. Intussusception. In: Grosfeld JL, O'Neill JA, Coran AG, Fonkalsrud EW, Caldamone AA, eds. *Pediatric Surgery.* 6th ed. Philadelphia, PA: Mosby Elsevier; 2006:1313–1341

Chapter 8

Newborn Hematemesis and Scrotal Swelling

Presentation

A 1-week-old boy is brought to the emergency department (ED) because of a single episode of vomiting brownish material that his parents think is blood. They have also noticed that his left testicle is swollen and purplish. The family has no doctor. The child has been breastfeeding well, except that mother has had some pain in her nipples from vigorous sucking. They bring in a blanket stained with brownish emesis.

Past medical history includes birth weight of 3.2 kg. The patient was born at term in a home birth attended by a nonmedical birth attendant. Apgar scores were 8 and 9.

Examination reveals the following vital signs: rectal temperature 37.3°C, pulse 110 beats/min, respiration 40 breaths/min, and blood pressure 90/50 mm Hg. He is well developed and nourished. Examination of head, eyes, ears, nose, and throat is negative for any signs of oral or nasal bleeding. His heartbeat is regular with no murmurs. His lungs are clear. His abdomen is soft and nontender. There are no inguinal hernias. His penis is uncircumcised. The left hemiscrotum is swollen and purplish in color, similar to a bruise. His right hemiscrotum appears to be normal. There are small bruises on both arms. Mongolian spots are visible over the back.

Discussion

Differential Diagnosis

- Hematemesis due to swallowed maternal blood (versus gastrointestinal bleeding)
- Scrotal hematocele
- Hemorrhagic diathesis

Evaluation

Laboratory evaluation is performed and guaiac of the brownish emesis is positive. Complete blood count reveals white blood cells 14,100/μL, 40% segmented neutrophils, 6% bands, 40% lymphocytes, 14% monocytes, hemoglobin 14 g/dL, hematocrit 42%, and platelet count 405,000/μL. Prothrombin time was 220 seconds and partial thromboplastin time, 50 seconds (both prolonged).

Apt test of the blood on the blanket is consistent with fetal blood.

Diagnosis is hemorrhagic disease of the newborn.

Treatment

This patient presents with 3 sites of bleeding: gastrointestinal, scrotum, and extremity bruising. These findings greatly increase the likelihood that a coagulopathy is present. However, in many newborns with hematemesis, the cause is benign, the result of swallowing blood during the birth process or while breastfeeding, with bleeding occurring from nipple fissures. This diagnosis is best evaluated by the Apt test, which distinguishes adult from fetal hemoglobin on the basis of denaturation of adult hemoglobin by alkali. In the case of swallowed blood, maternal adult hemoglobin will be identified on the blanket, instead of the infant's fetal hemoglobin.

The prothrombin time and partial thromboplastin time are both pro-longed. Administration of vitamin K corrects this within a few hours. More rapid correction can be achieved with intravenous fresh frozen plasma and intravenous vitamin K. The potential benefit of intravenous administration must be balanced against the risk of potentially life-threatening adverse reactions reported after intravenous vitamin K.

Keep in Mind

Patients without a primary care physician have less access to follow-up care and might depend on the ED for follow-up. There might be other reasons why they do not have a primary care physician that might complicate the social circumstances of their encounter.

Infants born at home may have reduced access to primary care. The involvement of nonmedical sources of primary care might place them at risk for unconventional illnesses that normal hospital nursery routines would usually prevent or identify early, such as ophthalmia neonatorum, hemorrhagic disease of the newborn, phenylketonuria, other inborn errors of metabolism, and congenital hypothyroidism.

Hemorrhagic disease of the newborn results from vitamin K deficiency. The absence of bacterial gut flora responsible for vitamin K synthesis at birth results in a delay in vitamin K synthesis. Limited stores can potentially be exhausted before gut flora synthesis of vitamin K ensues. Breast milk is a poor source of vitamin K. Routinely administered vitamin K in the nursery is an effective prophylactic measure against hemorrhagic disease of the newborn.

Recommended Reading

Stoll BJ. Blood disorders. In: Kliegman RM, Behrman RE, Jenson HB, Stanton BF, eds. *Nelson Textbook of Pediatrics.* 18th ed. Int ed. Philadelphia, PA: WB Saunders; 2007:766-774

Chapter 9

Constipation, Abdominal Pain, and Vomiting

Presentation

A 4-year-old previously healthy boy presents with constipation and abdominal pain of 2 days' duration and vomiting of 1 day's duration. The pain localizes to the periumbilical region and causes him to cry out intermittently. He has had multiple episodes of nonbloody emesis. His mother denies fevers, chills, and cough. He previously had regular bowel movements, and none of his stools were bloody. At another emergency department (ED), a dose of laxative provided no relief. His white blood cell (WBC) count is elevated and prompts transfer to your pediatric ED.

He is afebrile with normal vital signs. Although he seems sleepy, he is able to be aroused and exhibits age-appropriate behavior. Bowel sounds are hypoactive. His abdomen is not distended, but you note periumbilical tenderness and a right-sided mass. Rectal examination produces soft guaiac-negative stool.

Discussion

Differential Diagnosis
- Constipation
- Trauma, including inflicted injury
- Appendicitis
- Gastroenteritis
- Intussusception
- Intraabdominal or retroperitoneal neoplasm

Evaluation
Abdominal radiographs reveal a semilunate opacity in the right upper abdomen with no air fluid levels or significant paucity of bowel gas. Laboratory tests performed in your ED include WBC (20,500/µL), hemoglobin (12.4 g/dL), platelets (584,000/µL), and normal chemistry panel without acidosis.

Despite the guaiac-negative stool, the radiograph is suspicious for intussusception. A contrast enema reveals no evidence of intussusception, but a competent ileocecal valve prevents reflux into the terminal ileum. The patient tolerates oral intake, but reexamination reveals persisting abdominal discomfort. The subsequent computed tomography scan reveals the "target" sign of intussusception and no evidence of appendicitis or intraperitoneal fluid (figures 9-1 and 9-2). The patient subsequently begins to pass guaiac-positive, mucoid stools.

Treatment
Because his initial contrast enema encountered a competent ileocecal valve and failed to demonstrate the intussusception, further hydrostatic attempts at reduction are deemed futile. At laparotomy, unsuccessful manual reduction leads to resection of a segment of small bowel containing the ileoileal intussusception and a Meckel diverticulum.

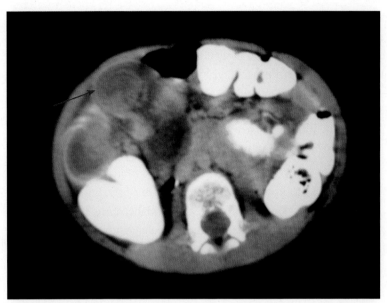

Figure 9-1

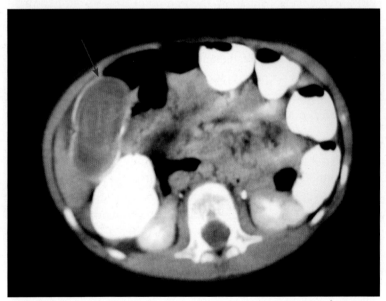

Figure 9-2

Keep in Mind

After constipation, intussusception is the most common cause of abdominal pain in infants and preschool-aged children. The cardinal symptoms are intermittent pain, vomiting, and bloody stool. Although severe colicky pain is the most common symptom, 15% to 20% may experience no pain. Vomiting is often the earliest symptom, but it may be absent in 30% to 40% of cases. The full triad of symptoms occurs together in only 10% of cases. Other misleading symptoms include fever in approximately 10% and diarrhea in 10% to 15% of cases.

Bloody stools and right upper quadrant mass have a high positive predictive value, but specific signs are often lacking. Furthermore, no individual clinical feature has excellent negative predictive value; the absence of rectal bleeding or right upper quadrant mass does not reliably exclude the diagnosis. Among patients with intussusception who do not have grossly bloody stool, 75% of cases may be positive for occult blood.

Most cases of intussusception are idiopathic and lack a pathologic lead point (PLP). In the typical situation, the lead point consists of thickened Peyer patches, which are abundant and often circumferential in the distal ileum. Pathologic lead points may be focal (eg, Meckel diverticulum, polyps, gastrointestinal duplications, malignancies such as lymphoma) or diffuse (eg, Henoch-Schönlein purpura, cystic fibrosis). The discovery of PLPs is more likely with increasing age, ileoileal or ileoileocolic intussusception, recurrent intussusception, and longer duration of symptoms.

Plain film abdominal radiographs may be normal in 30% of cases and may reveal a definite gas-outlined intussusception in only 15%. Clinical suspicion for intussusception may be more important in guiding therapy even if radiologic studies are nondiagnostic. Because most intussusception cases are ileocolic, they are amenable to detection and reduction by contrast or air enema. However, ileoileal intussusception or the ileoileal portion of an ileoileocolic intussusception may escape detection if the ileocecal valve does not permit reflux of contrast. Hence, clinical suspicion for intussusception must always remain high until the resolution of symptoms occurs.

Recommended Reading

Byrne AT, Geoghegan T, Govender P, Lyburn ID, Colhoun E, Torreggiani WC. The imaging of intussusception. *Clin Radiol.* 2005;60:39–46

Losek JD. Intussusception: don't miss the diagnosis! *Pediatr Emerg Care.* 1993;9:46–51

Losek JD, Fiete RL. Intussusception and the diagnostic value of testing stool for occult blood. *Am J Emerg Med.* 1991;9:1–3

Chapter 10

Diarrhea and Pallor

Presentation

A 12-month-old boy is brought to the emergency department because of
fussiness, diarrhea, and pale color. He became ill yesterday with 2 episodes
of diarrhea. Today, he has had 3 episodes of loose, watery stools. His color
is obviously pale. No fever or vomiting is present.

Past medical history is significant for mild prematurity; the baby was born
at 35 weeks' gestation. Birth weight was 2.7 kg. Apgar scores were 8 and 9.
He did well in the nursery and was discharged from the hospital on day
3 of life.

Examination reveals the following vital signs: rectal temperature 37.8°C,
pulse 130 beats/min, respiration 60 breaths/min, blood pressure 80/65 mm
Hg, and weight in the 25th percentile. Oxygen saturation is 75% in room
air. He is placed on oxygen by nonrebreather mask, and his oxygen saturation now reads 94%. He is active and fussy. His color is pale and he looks
ill. Examination of head, eyes, ears, nose, and throat is normal except for
facial pallor. Mucosa is moist; his neck is supple. His heartbeat is regular
with no murmur. You note that the lungs have clear aeration with moderate tachypnea and no retractions. His abdomen is soft with normal bowel
sounds. He moves all his extremities well. His extremities are warm but
pale. Capillary refill time is 4 seconds. One of the nurses describes his
color as grayish.

Discussion

Differential Diagnosis
- Hypoxemia
- Respiratory failure
- Anemia
- Poor skin perfusion
- Methemoglobinemia

Evaluation
Laboratory evaluation is performed with the following findings of arterial blood gas while breathing supplemental oxygen: pH 7.19, P_{CO_2} 25 mm Hg, P_{O_2} 380 mm Hg, base excess -17, oxygen saturation 100%, sodium 139 mmol/L, potassium 5.2 mmol/L, chloride 110 mmol/L, bicarbonate 7 mmol/L, and glucose 150 mg/dL. The resident reports that the color of the blood is brown, like a chocolate bar. The nurse confirms this bizarre finding.

Complete blood count reveals the following: white blood cells 16,100/μL, 50% segmented neutrophils, 10% bands, 40% lymphocytes, hemoglobin 12 g/dL, hematocrit 36%, and platelets 480,000/μL.

Chest radiograph reveals clear lung fields and a normal cardiac silhouette. Cooximetry was performed; methemoglobin level is 30% and oxygen saturation 70%. A glucose-6-phosphate dehydrogenase (G6PD) assay returns normal.

You diagnose the patient with methemoglobinemia.

Treatment
The patient is immediately treated by administering oxygen, infusing intravenous (IV) fluids, and reassessing his oxygen saturation, which continues to be low. He is then treated with IV methylene blue. His color improves dramatically, his methemoglobin levels decline, and his oxygen saturation improves.

A general principle in identifying respiratory failure is that the oxygen saturation should improve to 100% when supplemental oxygen is applied.

Nasal cannula oxygen increases the fraction of inspired oxygen (FIO_2) modestly. An oxygen mask can deliver a higher FIO_2. Nonrebreather oxygen masks with a good seal can deliver close to 100% FIO_2 at high oxygen flow rates. Very high FIO_2s should be able to overcome most pulmonary disease conditions to sufficiently oxygenate the patient. If the oxygen saturation is not 100% on a very high FIO_2, respiratory failure should be suspected and positive pressure respiratory support should be considered (eg, mask continuous positive airway pressure, bilevel positive airway pressure, tracheal intubation). However, in this case, the patient's respiratory effort and air exchange by auscultation are excellent. Additionally, his chest radiograph is normal. Thus, significant lung disease is unlikely the cause here.

Methemoglobin is immediately suspected. Typically, these patients manifest symptoms of gastroenteritis. Their skin color is classically described as ashen gray. If the methemoglobin level is high enough, the color of the blood will be chocolate brown. This is highly diagnostic if found, but in most cases, the methemoglobin level is not high enough for this finding to be dramatic.

Methemoglobin is an abnormal hemoglobin that does not carry or release oxygen (similar to carboxyhemoglobin in carbon monoxide poisoning). The cause of methemoglobinemia is often unclear. It can result from oxidative stress from drugs such as sulfonamides, phenazopyridine, and chemicals such as nitrates or nitrites. It usually resolves with a low risk of recurrence.

Pulse oximetry measures the oxygen saturation (percentage of hemoglobin molecules that are carrying oxygen) by measuring the light absorption at 2 wavelengths. The pulse oximeter probe has 2 light sources, a red and an infrared source. The red source is visible, but not the infrared source. By measuring absorption through the capillaries, the pulse oximeter calculates the oxygen saturation, essentially on the basis of color. The light absorption characteristics for saturated and desaturated adult hemoglobin A are known, and by measuring the differential light absorption, the pulse oximeter calculates the oxygen saturation percentage. Fetal hemoglobin (newborn) and sickle hemoglobin are not the same as adult hemoglobin A; however, their light absorption characteristics are similar to adult hemoglobin A, so oxygen saturation measurements via pulse oximetry are still reasonably accurate in newborns and in patients with sickle hemoglobin.

However, methemoglobin light absorption is significantly different from adult hemoglobin A. Fortunately, the oxygen saturation reads in the correct direction (ie, it reads a low oxygen saturation). In other words, a patient with methemoglobinemia will have a low oxygen saturation if measured by pulse oximetry, making the diagnosis more apparent. On the other hand, in carboxyhemoglobin (carbon monoxide poisoning), the oxygen saturation by pulse oximetry will read artificially high, making the identification of carbon monoxide poisoning more difficult.

Many references suggest the use of a bedside test to help confirm the presence of methemoglobinemia. This is done by obtaining a drop of blood from the patient and placing it onto a filter paper pad or gauze pad. The oxygen in room air should cause a dark blood sample containing normal hemoglobin to turn red. However, in methemoglobinemia, the color of the blood will remain unchanged. Although this test is commonly suggested, it does not yield any new information because pulse oximetry measurements will have already confirmed that the administration of oxygen results in only a modest increase in oxygen saturation. This visual test of checking for the color change of a blood sample was primarily used in the era before pulse oximetry.

Because methemoglobin cannot carry or deliver oxygen, the maximum oxygen saturation of a patient with 30% methemoglobin is only 70%. In the absence of preexisting pulmonary disease, the administration of supplemental oxygen will not change the maximal oxygen content. Your patient's initial oxygen saturation by pulse oximetry was 75%. Oxygen administration increased the reading to 94% by pulse oximetry. The oxygen saturation measured on the blood gas was 100%. The oxygen saturation by cooximetry was 70%. How can all these differences be reconciled?

Table 10-1 describes the oxygen saturation measurements by arterial blood gas analysis, pulse oximetry, and cooximetry for a normal patient breathing room air and a patient with 30% methemoglobin breathing room air.

Table 10-1. Saturation Measurements for a Normal Patient Breathing Room Air and a Patient With 30% Methemoglobin Breathing Room Air

Breathing Room Air	Normal, Hemoglobin = 12.0 g/dL	30% Methemoglobin, Hemoglobin = 12.0 g/dL
Po_2	100 mm Hg	100 mm Hg
Oxygen saturation by arterial blood gas analysis	99%	99%
Oxygen saturation by pulse oximetry	99%	75%
Oxygen saturation by cooximetry	99%	69%
Oxygenated hemoglobin content	11.9 g/dL	8.3 g/dL

The Po_2 reflects the gas tension of dissolved oxygen, resulting from diffusion of oxygen through alveoli and capillaries. For example, the Po_2 in room air is 160 mm Hg (760 mm Hg times 21% Fio_2). Thus, a cup of water sitting on a desk has a Po_2 of 160 mm Hg (simple gas diffusion). This Po_2 is higher than that of the blood, but the oxygen content of the cup of water is very low, whereas the oxygen content of blood is much higher. The Po_2 measures gas tension, not oxygen content.

We know that the normal oxygen-hemoglobin dissociation curve looks like Figure 10-1. At a Po_2 of 80 mm Hg, hemoglobin should be 96% saturated. At a Po_2 of 100 mm Hg, hemoglobin should be 99% saturated. This curve is programmed into the blood gas machine. The blood gas analyzer does not measure the oxygen saturation; rather, it is calculated on the basis of this curve. A blood gas analyzer assumes the sample contains a normal blood sample containing hemoglobin A, and uses the hemoglobin A oxygen-hemoglobin dissociation curve to calculate the oxygen saturation. In a patient with methemoglobinemia, a significant portion of hemoglobin is not normal hemoglobin A, which is why the oxygen saturation determined by the blood gas analyzer is incorrect. Pulse oximetry measures oxygen saturation by using light absorption. However, light

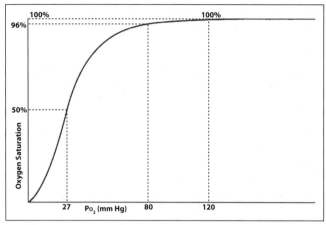

Figure 10-1

absorption values are optimized for adult hemoglobin A. In methemo-globinemia, the oxygen saturation measured by pulse oximetry is not correct, but at least it still reads low. Cooximetry uses 4 or more light sources so it can more accurately determine true hemoglobin oxygen saturation. Light absorption data from 4 light wavelength sources permit more mathematical equations to derive the oxygen saturation of adult hemoglobin A, methemoglobin, and carboxyhemoglobin.

In Table 10-2, the oxygen saturation measurements for blood gas, pulse oximetry, and cooximetry are all correct for adult hemoglobin A. However, for methemoglobin, only the cooximetry measurement is accurate. Once the patient is on supplemental oxygen, the oxygen saturation data potentially change (Table 10-2).

The patient is breathing high-flow oxygen. The gas tension of oxygen is high, but the oxygen content and saturation change very little. The blood gas analyzer measures a Po_2 of 380 mm Hg and it reports that the oxygen saturation should be 100% at this Po_2 because it assumes that the sample contains adult hemoglobin A. Interestingly, the oxygen saturation by pulse oximetry rises even in the patient with the methemoglobin, probably because of a mixture of the different hemoglobins and the rising saturation of hemoglobin A. Cooximetry measures the correct oxygen saturation.

Table 10-2. Oxygen Saturation Measurements for Blood Gas, Pulse Oximetry, and Cooximetry

Breathing High Flow O_2	Normal, Hemoglobin = 12.0 g/dL	30% Methemoglobin, Hemoglobin = 12.0 g/dL
Po_2	380 mm Hg	380 mm Hg
Oxygen saturation by arterial blood gas analysis	100%	100%
Oxygen saturation by pulse oximetry	100%	94%
Oxygen saturation by cooximetry	100%	70%
Oxygenated hemoglobin content	12.0 g/dL	8.4 g/dL

Some medical centers routinely perform cooximetry on all blood gas samples, so it is important for clinicians to know whether the oxygen saturation value on a blood gas is simply a calculated value from the blood gas analyzer or a measured value from a cooximeter.

Keep in Mind

The main clinical consequence of significant methemoglobin levels is that it reduces oxygen-carrying capacity. A patient with a hemoglobin of 12 g/dL and 30% methemoglobin has the equivalent normal hemoglobin of only 8.4 g/dL. This is not immediately life threatening, but it reduces tissue oxygenation. For patients who are more anemic, the effects of methemoglobinemia would be more severe. Although oxygen-carrying capacity is acutely reduced, the cardiovascular system can partially compensate by increasing the cardiac output, which effectively increases the total oxygen delivery rate to the tissues. The reason for the metabolic acidosis in this case is partially bicarbonate loss from diarrhea and partially lactic acidosis due to inadequate tissue oxygen delivery (dehydration and methemoglobinemia).

Patients with modest degrees of methemoglobin can be treated with supplemental oxygen and IV fluid hydration. More severe degrees of methemoglobinemia can be treated with IV methylene blue. The biochemistry of this reaction is beyond the scope of this chapter. However, G6PD deficiency must be ruled out before methylene blue therapy is initiated.

Recommended Reading

Cohen AR, Manno CS. Hematologic emergencies. In: Fleisher GR, Ludwig S, Henretig FM, Ruddy RM, Silverman BK, eds. *Textbook of Pediatric Emergency Medicine.* 5th ed. Philadelphia, PA: Lippincott Williams & Wilkins; 2006:921–949

King BR, King C, Coates WC. Pulse oximetry. Critical procedures. In: Gausche-Hill M, Fuchs S, Yamamoto L, eds. *APLS: The Pediatric Emergency Medicine Resource.* 4th rev ed. Sudbury, MA: Jones and Bartlett Publishers; 2007:683–685

Yamamoto LG. Interpretation of blood gases and pulse oximetry. In: Yamamoto LG, Inaba AS, Okamoto JK, Patronis ME, Yamashiroya VK, eds. *Case Based Pediatrics for Medical Students and Residents.* Honolulu, HI: University of Hawaii; 2004:273–276. Available at: http://www.hawaii. edu/medicine/pediatrics/pedtext. Accessed December 10, 2008

Chapter 11

Nausea, Vomiting, and Headache

Presentation

A 17-year-old girl is brought to the emergency department (ED) by her older sister because of nausea, 5 episodes of vomiting, and headache for 14 hours. It is the winter flu season, and it has been snowing for the past 2 days. She denies diarrhea, dysuria, fever, or neck pain. Her last menstrual period was 2.5 months ago. She took a home pregnancy test 3 weeks ago that she thinks was positive, but the test result was unclear to her. She has not seen an obstetrician. She has not informed her parents of this possible pregnancy, and she requests that her parents not be notified.

Past medical history is negative.

Examination reveals the following vital signs: oral temperature 37.0°C, pulse 88 beats/min, respiration 14 breaths/min, blood pressure 110/60 mm Hg, and oxygen saturation 100% in room air. She is subdued but cooperative and alert. Fundi are normal. Pupils are reactive. Oral mucosa is moist. Her neck is supple. Her heartbeat is regular with no murmurs. Her lungs are clear. Her abdomen is flat and nontender with active bowel sounds. Her color and perfusion are good. Fetal heart tones cannot be detected.

Discussion

Differential Diagnosis
- Viral infection
- Gastroenteritis
- Hyperemesis gravidarum
- Carbon monoxide poisoning

Evaluation
An obstetrics consultation is obtained. The diagnostic impression is hyperemesis gravidarum without dehydration.

Treatment
A urine pregnancy test is positive. The obstetrician recommends telephone follow-up for tonight and office follow-up in 2 days, or return to the ED if her condition worsens.

Five hours after she is discharged from the ED, 2 nieces and a nephew of our patient who live in the same house are brought to the ED with similar symptoms. Carbon monoxide poisoning is suspected. Oxygen saturation by pulse oximetry is 100% in room air. An arterial blood gas on the sickest patient shows (in room air) pH 7.33, Pco_2 35 mm Hg, Po_2 100 mm Hg, base excess -7, and oxygen saturation 99%. However, cooximetry on the same blood sample shows oxygen saturation of 70%, and the carboxyhemoglobin level is 30%. The home is called to talk to the first patient, but there is no answer. According to relatives, she should be at home. The police are called, and they enter the house, only to find the patient extremely lethargic and weak. She is brought to the ED. She is immediately transferred to a hyperbaric oxygen facility, where she recovers. Six months later, she delivers a baby boy with severe neurologic impairment.

The diagnosis is carbon monoxide poisoning with fetal hypoxia.

Keep in Mind
This case presents the conflicting issues of confidentiality and parental consent for the care of minors. Although the patient is a minor, nearly all states have provisions that permit minors to consent for care on their own

(without parents) for reproductive health and substance abuse. Because she is requesting confidentiality, her parents cannot be notified without her consent.

Carbon monoxide poisoning cannot be detected by conventional pulse oximetry because it will read falsely high. An arterial blood gas measurement without cooximetry cannot definitively confirm it either. The oxygen saturation on the blood gas is calculated (not measured) on the basis of normal hemoglobin. The blood gas analyzer measures oxygen gas tension in millimeters of mercury; it then calculates what the oxygen saturation should be on the basis of the oxygen-hemoglobin dissociation curve (see Chapter 10). For the 2 wavelengths of light that the pulse oximeter uses, carboxyhemoglobin light absorption characteristics result in a falsely high pulse oximetry oxygen saturation. Carbon monoxide binds onto hemoglobin resulting in carboxyhemoglobin, which does not carry and release oxygen, basically rendering it useless. The only way to detect carbon monoxide poisoning is by measuring a carboxyhemoglobin level or by using a cooximeter, which reads oxygen saturation using 4 or more wavelengths (rather than the 2 wavelengths used by pulse oximetry) or by using multiple-light-source pulse oximetry (known as Masimo Rainbow technology). The last method is not routinely available in most medical centers at the time of this writing; however, its use is likely to increase in the future.

The diagnosis of carbon monoxide poisoning should be suspected in cold climates where fuel combustion heating is used. Wood-burning or coal-burning sources of heat are likely to emit carbon monoxide. Commercially manufactured fuel combustion heating units (eg, propane, natural gas, fuel oil) are designed to provide heat without carbon monoxide risk; however, if these units malfunction and do not combust fuel completely or if exhaust systems malfunction, carbon monoxide production is still possible. Automobile exhaust contains significant amounts of carbon monoxide. House fires pose significant risks of smoke inhalation as well as carbon monoxide risk. Cigarette smokers typically have carboxyhemoglobin levels of 5% to 10%.

Carboxyhemoglobinemia (carbon monoxide poisoning) is similar to methemoglobinemia in that both of these hemoglobins do not deliver oxygen to the tissues. However, carbon monoxide poisoning is more difficult to diagnose because patients look pink (classically, cherry red) compared with methemoglobinemia patients, who look pale or ashen gray. Conventional pulse oximetry reads low in methemoglobinemia, but it reads falsely high in carbon monoxide poisoning. Table 11-1 illustrates the differences in oxygenation parameters for a patient with a hemoglobin of 12.0 g/dL.

The immediate treatment for carbon monoxide poisoning is 100% oxygen. This can be achieved with a tight-fitting nonrebreather mask. The half-life of carboxyhemoglobin is approximately 4 hours in room air, but

Table 11-1. Differences in Oxygenation Parameters

Measurement	Normal Patient	30% Methemoglobin	30% Carboxyhemoglobin
Breathing room air			
Po_2	100 mm Hg	100 mm Hg	100 mm Hg
Oxygen saturation by arterial blood gas analysis	99%	99%	99%
Oxygen saturation by pulse oximetry	99%	75%	100%
Oxygen saturation by cooximetry	99%	69%	69%
Oxygenated hemoglobin content	11.9 g/dL	8.3 g/dL	8.3 g/dL
Breathing high-flow oxygen			
Po_2	300 mm Hg	300 mm Hg	300 mm Hg
Oxygen saturation by arterial blood gas analysis	100%	100%	100%
Oxygen saturation by pulse oximetry	100%	94%	100%
Oxygen saturation by cooximetry	100%	70%	70%
Oxygenated hemoglobin content	11.9 g/dL	8.4 g/dL	8.4 g/dL

this decreases to 1 hour if breathing pure oxygen and 30 minutes if breathing hyperbaric oxygen. Hyperbaric oxygen therapy should be considered for carbon monoxide poisoning.

Concomitant cyanide poisoning should also be considered.

Recommended Reading

Ewald MB, Baum CR. Environmental emergencies. In: Fleisher GR, Ludwig S, Henretig FM, Ruddy RM, Silverman BK, eds. *Textbook of Pediatric Emergency Medicine.* 5th ed. Philadelphia, PA: Lippincott Williams & Wilkins; 2006:1009–1031

King BR, King C, Coates WC. Pulse oximetry. Critical procedures. In: Gausche-Hill M, Fuchs S, Yamamoto L, eds. *APLS: The Pediatric Emergency Medicine Resource.* 4th rev ed. Sudbury, MA: Jones and Bartlett Publishers; 2007:683–685

Yamamoto LG. Interpretation of blood gases and pulse oximetry. In: Yamamoto LG, Inaba AS, Okamoto JK, Patronis ME, Yamashiroya VK, eds. *Case Based Pediatrics for Medical Students and Residents.* Honolulu, HI: University of Hawaii; 2004:273–276. Available at: http://www.hawaii.edu/medicine/pediatrics/pedtext. Accessed December 10, 2008

Chapter 12

Abdominal Pain and Adolescent Patient Confidentiality

Presentation

A 16-year-old girl is brought to the emergency department (ED) for abdominal pain. Her mother is concerned about the possibility of appendicitis because she walks very slowly and is hunched over as a result of pain. There is a history of fever (feeling warm), but no temperatures were measured at home. She has some mild nausea, but no vomiting or diarrhea. Her appetite is less, but she is taking in fluids and her urine output is good. There is no history of coughing, sore throat, or nasal congestion. Her last menstrual period was 5 weeks ago, but she states that she is often irregular.

Past medical history is negative.

Examination reveals the following vital signs: oral temperature 37.1°C, pulse 75 beats/min, respiration 18 breaths/min, blood pressure 100/75 mm Hg, and oxygen saturation 99% in room air. She is alert and cooperative and in no distress lying down. Examination of head, eyes, ears, nose, and throat is negative. Her heartbeat is regular with no murmurs. Her lungs are clear. Her abdomen is flat with some voluntary guarding. There is significant tenderness in the right upper quadrant and both lower quadrants. Her left upper quadrant is only minimally tender. Rebound tenderness is present over all 4 quadrants. Bowel sounds are normoactive. There is no flank tenderness, but this maneuver does result in some pelvic pain. There are no inguinal hernias. When asked to cough, she experiences moderately severe pain.

Discussion

Differential Diagnosis
- Appendicitis
- Pelvic inflammatory disease
- Mesenteric adenitis

Evaluation
The patient is offered narcotic analgesics; however, she chooses plain acetaminophen instead.

Her mother is asked to leave the room to complete the history. During this portion of the interview, the patient indicates that she has had sexual intercourse several times during the past year, with one sexual partner. She specifically requests that her mother not be told about this. They have been using condoms sometimes, but not always. She is not using any other contraception measures.

A pelvic examination is performed. The external examination is unremarkable. A speculum examination reveals a purulent discharge from the cervical os. Endocervix swabs for gonorrhea and chlamydia studies are sent for analysis. A bimanual examination reveals severe cervical motion tenderness and bilateral adnexal tenderness. No masses are palpable. A urine pregnancy test is negative.

The patient is informed that she probably has pelvic inflammatory disease (PID). Laboratory studies and a pelvic ultrasound are ordered. She asks how and why PID occurs. When she is told that this usually starts with a sexually transmitted infection, she immediately requests that her mother not be told.

Treatment
In most states, minors (the lower age limit varies, but it is usually about 14 years) can consent for medical care on their own for health or medical conditions related to substance abuse and reproductive health conditions. Because PID is a reproductive health condition, the patient can consent to care on her own. A parent's consent is not required. Because the teen can consent on her own, she also has the right to confidentiality.

Adolescents present some difficult issues with regard to consent and confidentiality. If a minor teen arrives in the ED with a complaint related to substance abuse or reproductive health, a registration clerk might automatically call the teen's parents to obtain consent for treatment. However, consent is not required in this instance, and it violates confidentiality. Alternatively, some teens might not desire confidentiality, and they might not fully understand medical care instructions without an adult parent. Medical complications could result if proper care instructions are not followed.

Confidentiality is difficult, perhaps impossible, to maintain when using many medical insurance programs. Generally, the subscriber to the medical insurance (usually an adult parent) is provided with all medical care statements that were paid by the medical insurance plan. These statements are usually itemized, so parents can easily determine that their teen was seen in the ED on a certain date and that some tests, including pregnancy and tests for sexually transmitted infections, were done. Thus, if a teen requests total information confidentiality, the parents' medical insurance information must be removed from the patient encounter. It is difficult, perhaps impossible, for a medical care provider, be it a doctor or hospital, to absolutely assure a teen patient of confidentiality when their parents' medical insurance is used because providers cannot reliably block parental notification. Additionally, parents deserve the right of awareness if their insurance plan is used.

This teen patient is provided with some counseling. She is told that it is not possible to ensure complete confidentiality of this information because she is using her mother's medical insurance. The teen has 4 options. First, she can tell her mother everything so that daughter and parent can take care of this medical condition together. Second, the teen patient can waive confidentiality (ie, she can consent to disclosure of all medical information), thus permitting the physician to discuss the teen's condition with her mother. This strategy lets the doctor break the news to the mother. Third, the teen patient can maintain confidentiality, but then she must remove her mother's medical insurance information from the encounter, in which case the teen will be responsible for the bill. Bills will be addressed to the teen at her mailing address. If this is her parents' home address, then it is possible that her parents could open her mail. A third-party address (eg, a friend's, an aunt's) could also be used. Finally, the teen patient can maintain confidentiality for now but permit the transfer of the medical insurance claim information. This is essentially a waiver of confidentiality as it relates to the medical insurance claim information. By consenting to this, the teen must consent to the likelihood that the hospital's medical insurance claim information will be disclosed to her parents.

Although some might consider these 4 options to be coercive, this is simply advising teens who are capable of making these important decisions for themselves. They should be helped through this process. The complexities of submitting medical insurance claims make this process difficult to guarantee confidentiality. For emergency care in particular, it is possible that at least 4 separate claims will be submitted, one each for physician services, hospital services, laboratory services, and pharmacy services. Additionally, the involvement of a radiologist or other medical consultants will result in additional claims. Preventing all of these claims from reaching the teen's parents is beyond what an ED physician can guarantee.

During additional counseling, our patient is advised that because her mother is here, she will ask about her daughter's diagnosis, and she will ask other obvious questions. If the doctor cannot answer her mother's questions to maintain confidentiality, then her mother will ask her daughter these questions. In other instances, when parents are not with their teens when they visit the ED, teens should understand that purchasing medication without medical insurance is very expensive, and the complexity of following medical instructions is a difficult task without parental support. Some teens who are making such important decisions on their own for the first time will generally consent to informing their parents. Teens might choose to tell their mothers everything, or have the care provider tell the mothers on the teens' behalf. Their choice (ie, to what they are consenting) must be clearly documented in the medical record.

This teen patient chooses to have the care provider tell her mother on her behalf. The physician has a discussion with her mother, who is advised of the importance of a supportive parental presence at this time.

A serum beta human chorionic gonadotropin test is negative. A pelvic ultrasound does not reveal any masses or abscesses. A complete blood count is normal. Liver enzymes are slightly increased.

The patient is diagnosed with PID and Fitz-Hugh-Curtis syndrome (perihepatitis) and treated with antibiotics.

Keep in Mind

Teens present challenges in simultaneously fulfilling consent and confidentiality requirements. The role of parents is important, but confidentiality requirements and the ability of minors to consent to care on their own (without parents) in specific circumstances require that emergency and primary care practitioners potentially rely on the decision-making capacity and the medical care responsibilities of teens. In most instances, the involvement of a parent in the care of a teen results in more mature decision-making, shared responsibility, and a greater degree of reliability in following through with medical plans and recommendations. However, when confidentiality is requested, this must be respected. There are also occasions when parents are abusive and nonsupportive, prompting teens to seek medical care and consent on their own. Although confidentiality is often desirable, physicians should advise teens of the many disadvantages of maintaining confidentiality. These include withholding important information from parents, the inability to use their parents' medical insurance, and the difficulty of reliably maintaining total confidentiality once patients leave the ED. In many instances, teens will waive confidentiality because parental involvement is preferable.

Recommended Reading

Selbst SM, DePiero AO. Medical-legal considerations. In: Gausche-Hill M, Fuchs S, Yamamoto L, eds. *APLS: The Pediatric Emergency Medicine Resource.* 4th rev ed. Sudbury, MA: Jones and Bartlett Publishers; 2007:610–637

Chapter 13

Long-standing Painless Abdominal Mass

Presentation

The family of this 34-month-old girl has noticed an abdominal protuber-ance for 2 months. However, she has continued to appear well without fever, systemic symptoms, abdominal pain, vomiting, or diarrhea. Her behavior and play continued without disturbance. During a routine physi-cal examination, detection of the mass prompts referral to your emergency department for further evaluation. She has had no bowel or bladder dys-function, nor has she had any abnormalities of gait, strength, or balance. She is alert, interactive, and well perfused, with normal vital signs. A large, firm, nontender mass has arisen in the center of the abdomen, with no distention or organomegaly (figures 13-1 and 13-2). No adenopathy or masses are present elsewhere. There is no nystagmus or opsoclonus. She has normal, symmetrical tone and strength. She has no petechiae, purpura, or bruising.

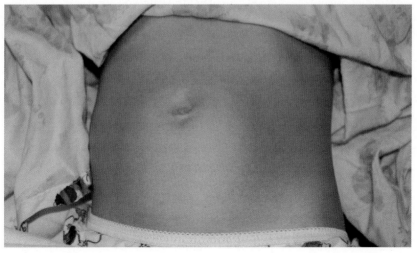

Figure 13-1

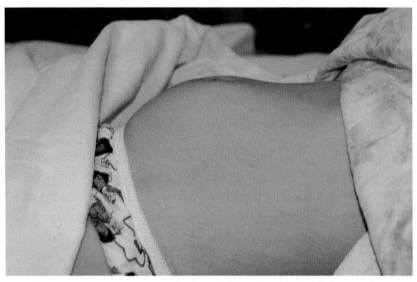

Figure 13-2

Discussion

Differential Diagnosis
- Bowel obstruction or other intraluminal distention
- Intraperitoneal fluid
- Isolated organ enlargement (eg, hepatomegaly, splenomegaly, hydronephrosis)
- Pancreatic pseudocyst
- Malignancy (eg, Wilms tumor, neuroblastoma, lymphoma)
- Other neoplasm (teratoma)
- Infection (eg, abscess, mycobacterial disease)
- Intestinal pathology (eg, duplication, fecal mass, pancreatic pseudocyst)

Evaluation
Abdominal radiographs reveal a large, calcified midabdominal mass (Figure 13-3). Blood studies include the following results: white blood cell count 12,300/µL with normal differential, hemoglobin 12.5 g/dL, platelet count 324,000/µL, normal electrolytes and transaminases, and lactate dehydrogenase 893 U/L.

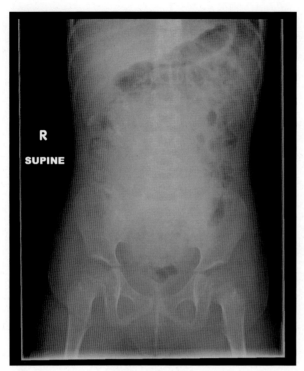

Figure 13-3

Treatment

Although Wilms tumor initially seems likely on the basis of the lack of systemic symptoms, the calcification suggests a neuroblastoma or, remotely, an extremely large teratoma. The patient is kept fasting with intravenous fluids containing no potassium until the risk of tumor lysis is excluded. The oncology service admits her for further evaluation with imaging and surgical consultation. Computed tomography (CT) imaging reveals a large (10 × 9 × 12 cm) heterogeneous abdominal mass that contains fluid, coarse calcifications, and fat (Figure 13-4). Its origin is uncertain, but CT reveals no local invasion, spinal involvement, or evidence of metastatic spread. The remainder of her tumor evaluation is unremarkable, with normal levels of alpha-fetoprotein, human chorionic gonadotropin, and urinary catecholamines.

After the medical evaluation reveals no evidence of malignancy, the patient undergoes surgical exploration, right oophorectomy, and excision of a large right adnexal mass with histopathology consistent with a mature cystic teratoma, a benign tumor requiring no further treatment once removed.

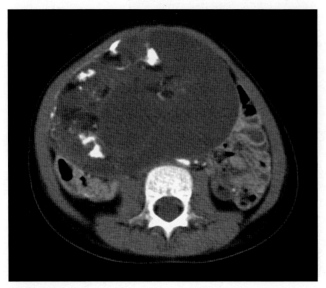

Figure 13-4

Keep in Mind

A long-standing abdominal mass in childhood is concerning for the possibility of malignancy. Masses can grow to impressive sizes without causing symptoms or prompting the family to seek medical care.

Although adnexal masses are often painless, they may become symptomatic when associated with torsion.

Recommended Reading

Avner JR. Abdominal distension. In: Fleisher GR, Ludwig S, Henretig FM, Ruddy RM, Silverman BK. *Textbook of Pediatric Emergency Medicine.* 5th ed. Philadelphia, PA: Lippincott Williams & Wilkins; 2006:175–181

Part 2

Febrile Illnesses

Chapter 14

Fever and Abdominal Pain

Presentation

A previously healthy 5-year-old girl presents with fever and abdominal pain of 1 day's duration. No vomiting, diarrhea, or dysuria is present. She initially experienced right-sided back pain, which spread to both sides of the back. She points to her entire abdomen when asked about the source of pain. There is no history of trauma. She is initially afebrile (36.8°C) but tachycardic (152 beats/min). Her perfusion is normal, and she is able to walk without a limp or any apparent worsening of abdominal pain. She has diffuse abdominal tenderness that does not localize to any quadrant, and she exhibits no guarding. She complains of worsened pain with jarring movements of the pelvis. No rash is present.

Discussion

Differential Diagnosis
- Urinary tract infection or pyelonephritis
- Diabetes mellitus
- Appendicitis
- Psoas abscess
- Gastroenteritis
- Osteomyelitis (vertebral or pelvic)

Evaluation
Urinalysis is positive (1+) for leukocyte esterase, but the patient's urine sediment contains only 10 to 20 white blood cells (WBC) per high-powered field. Urinary infection alone should not account for the type of pain the

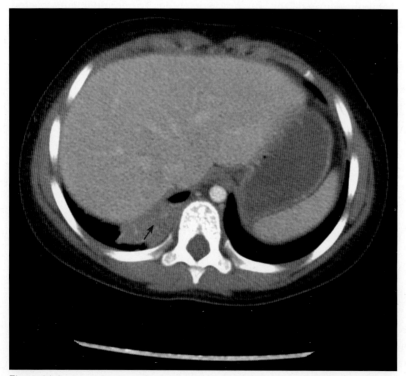

Figure 14-1

patient is experiencing. She receives an intravenous (IV) fluid bolus and an analgesic while awaiting the results of diagnostic tests.

The results of the diagnostic tests include the following: WBC 18,300/µL with normal differential and C-reactive protein 7.9 mg/dL. While under observation, her temperature increases to 41.0°C and she is provided acetaminophen. Although she now states that she feels better, her abdomen remains diffusely tender. She undergoes an IV-contrast-enhanced computed tomography (CT) scan of her abdomen and pelvis.

After she returns from the CT suite, the patient claims that she is now free of pain. She is able to walk without any difficulty, and her fever has resolved. CT scan shows no evidence of appendicitis, but a right lower lobe consolidation suggests pneumonia (Figure 14-1).

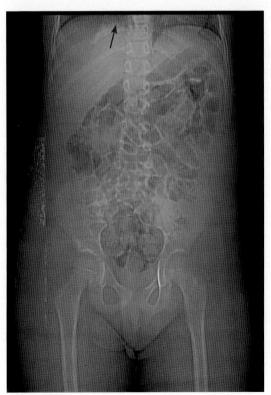

Figure 14-2

Treatment

Repeat examination of the chest after knowledge of the CT results reveals no obvious evidence of pneumonia. Nonetheless, the clinical course is consistent with an occult pneumonia. Retrospective review of the scout film reveals an infiltrate hidden behind the right hemidiaphragm (Figure 14-2). Therefore, the patient receives ceftriaxone 50 mg/kg IV followed by high-dose amoxicillin. She recovers without complications.

Keep in Mind

Pneumonia can manifest in a misleading fashion with fever and abdominal pain with or without localizing tenderness or suggestive respiratory symptoms or findings. Plain radiography of the chest, or even of the abdomen, is not appropriate for the majority of cases of abdominal pain. However, a chest radiograph may be useful in the case of unexplained high fever and poorly localizing abdominal pain. The upper portion of an abdominal film occasionally reveals pneumonia to be the cause of abdominal pain.

Pyuria should not prompt dismissal of abdominal pain as mere urinary infection when there are significant abdominal complaints or findings.

Despite the availability of laboratory testing and radiography, clinical examination and suspicion along with serial examinations are the most important tools in the initial evaluation of abdominal pain.

Recommended Reading

Kanegaye JT, Harley JR. Pneumonia in unexpected locations: an occult cause of pediatric abdominal pain. *J Emerg Med.* 1995;13:773–779

Chapter 15

Prolonged Fever Without Obvious Source

Presentation

A 4-year-old girl is brought to the emergency department because she has been experiencing temperatures as high as 41°C for 9 days with vomiting, abdominal pain, and mild cough and rhinorrhea. She has vomited once or twice a day and complains of left-sided abdominal pain that is worse when she walks. Urinary frequency and dysuria occur occasionally. Two days ago, her primary care physician prescribed trimethoprim-sulfamethoxazole for a possible urinary infection. Because of lack of response to the antibiotic, her physician ordered radiographs and blood tests. You review the results—white blood cell count 28,600/μL, erythrocyte sedimentation rate 72 mm/h, and no serologic evidence of mycoplasma or Epstein-Barr virus infection. Chest radiography reveals a subtle left lower lobe atelectasis but no consolidation. A urine sample yields no bacterial growth to date.

She is alert and well perfused. Her temperature is 38.6°C, but otherwise her vital signs are normal, including blood pressure of 98/55 mm Hg. She has clear, unlabored respirations and a soft, nontender anterior abdomen with normal bowel sounds. Her left flank is mildly and inconsistently tender. No masses are palpable. There is no spinous or costovertebral angle tenderness, and external genitalia are normal.

Discussion

Differential Diagnosis

- Viral infection (either a single prolonged illness or sequential infections)
- Pyelonephritis
- Pneumonia
- Intraabdominal abscess
- Skeletal infection
- Rheumatologic disease (eg, juvenile idiopathic arthritis)
- Inflammatory bowel disease
- Drug reaction/drug fever
- Malignancy (eg, leukemia, lymphoma)
- Unusual bacterial infections (eg, brucellosis, rickettsial diseases, enteric fever)

Evaluation

Although there is no clinical evidence for peritoneal irritation, you obtain a computed tomography (CT) scan of the abdomen and pelvis because of the patient's prolonged fever and abdominal complaints. According to the initial after-hours interpretation, the CT reveals no abscess or evidence of intraabdominal inflammation, but it does show the previously identified atelectasis. There is no other evidence for a serious bacterial focus or risk of clinical deterioration. Therefore, despite the absence of a proven diagnosis, you feel that she is a suitable candidate for outpatient observation.

Treatment

Despite the absence of demonstrated focus of infection or inflammation, the markedly elevated inflammatory indices prompt concern for an occult, deep-seated bacterial infection. Based on this concern, the patient receives ceftriaxone 50 mg/kg intravenously before discharge. She is instructed to continue her present medications and to follow up with her primary physician in 1 or 2 days. Later the same day, the radiology department calls to report the additional finding of a wedge-shaped, nonenhancing lucency in the upper pole of the left kidney (figures 15-1 and 15-2). On the basis of this finding, you make arrangements with her primary care practitioner for

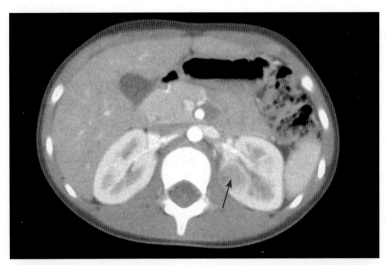

Figure 15-1

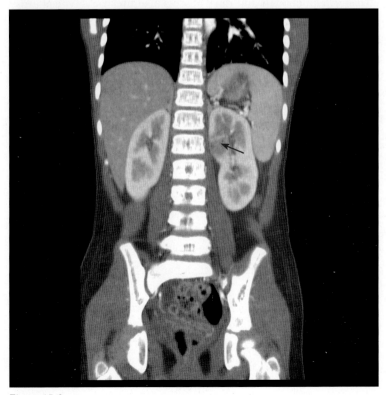

Figure 15-2

the patient to receive outpatient treatment for acute focal bacterial nephritis (lobar nephronia), consisting of daily injections of ceftriaxone in the office until afebrile, followed by oral antibiotics.

Clinical resolution is rapid, and a follow-up ultrasound 6 weeks later reveals resolution of the renal changes with no abscess or enlargement.

Keep in Mind

Acute focal bacterial nephritis (formerly called acute lobar nephronia because of its resemblance to pneumonia) is an increasingly recognized condition. The appearance on ultrasound is that of a focal mass with irregular borders, in contrast to a renal abscess, which has a hypoechoic or anechoic center with a well-defined border. Computed tomography imaging reveals the lesion to be a wedge-shaped, poorly defined region of decreased density. Acute focal bacterial nephritis likely represents an intermediate stage between pyelonephritis and renal abscess. Cultures yield typical uropathogens, although nearly 25% of the results from urine cultures may be negative. The optimal management is not established, but 3-week sequential parenteral-oral antibiotic courses may be more successful than 2-week courses.

Recommended Reading

Cheng CH, Tsau YK, Hsu SY, Lee TL. Effective ultrasonographic predictor for the diagnosis of acute lobar nephronia. *Pediatr Infect Dis J.* 2004;23:11–14

Cheng CH, Tsau YK, Lin TY. Effective duration of antimicrobial therapy for the treatment of acute lobar nephronia. *Pediatrics.* 2006;117:e84–e89

Klar A, Hurvitz H, Berkun Y, et al. Focal bacterial nephritis (lobar nephronia) in children. *J Pediatr.* 1996;128:850–853

Rathore MH, Barton LL, Luisiri A. Acute lobar nephronia: a review. *Pediatrics.* 1991;87:728–734

Seidel T, Kuwertz-Broking E, Kaczmarek S, et al. Acute focal bacterial nephritis in 25 children. *Pediatr Nephrol.* 2007;22:1897–1901

Chapter 16

Fever and Extensive Bruising

Presentation

A 13-year-old girl is brought to the emergency department with a chief complaint of fever. An acetaminophen tablet was provided that lowered her temperature; however, the fever returned 4 hours later. She has a slight cough and nasal congestion. She has experienced no vomiting, diarrhea, or headache. Appetite is somewhat lessened, with good fluid intake. Urine output is normal and she has not experienced dysuria. She denies taking ibuprofen or other nonsteroidal antiinflammatory medications.

Past medical history is negative.

Examination reveals the following vital signs: tympanic temperature 38.1°C, pulse 90 beats/min, respiration 18 breaths/min, and oxygen saturation 100% in room air. She is alert and active, in no distress. Her eyes are clear. Tympanic membranes are normal. There is mild clear mucus rhinorrhea congestion. Her pharynx is normal. Her neck is supple, without adenopathy. Heart, lung, and abdomen examinations are normal. Her skin examination is normal except for her back (Figure 16-1). There is extensive bruising over her back with some petechiae along these bruises. However, no bruising or petechiae are found elsewhere.

Her mother is asked how her daughter got these bruises. Her mother replies that she scraped her back with a coin to help to relieve the fever.

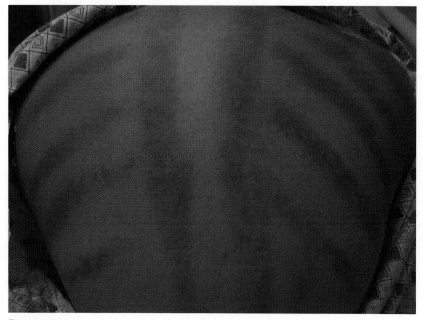

Figure 16-1

Discussion

Differential Diagnosis
- Fever with nonspecific findings
- Viral infection

Evaluation
The patient's extensive bruising is probably the result of coining, a routine practice in some cultures. A coin is used to scrape the skin until redness and bruising appear. The belief is that this increases blood flow to the skin to help reduce the fever.

Treatment
No additional treatment is needed for this patient and she is discharged with fever control instructions.

Keep in Mind

Coining should not be considered child abuse. Although it is an inflicted bruise, it is a cultural practice for some and it is not associated with more serious injuries such as fractures, brain injury, or death.

The pattern of coining can be linear, as in Figure 16-1 (a pattern that is consistent with coining), or it can be circular in shape with multiple circular bruises.

Cupping is another cultural practice in which negative pressure is applied with a suction cup, resulting in a suction bruise. In many instances, the cup is hot and inverted onto the skin. As the cup cools, it creates negative pressure. This results in circular suction bruises and the heat may result in burns on the circumference of the bruise.

Moxibustion is a practice linked to acupuncture in which incense is burned over a strategic area of the body. This can result in superficial burns resembling cigarette burns.

A visible bruising pattern that is inconsistent with coining, cupping, or suction bruises should be assumed to be ecchymosis, purpura, or petechiae. Patients should be evaluated for medical conditions such as coagulopathy, thrombocytopenia, platelet dysfunction, or vasculitis. A report to child protective services should be made if the bruising pattern suggests an inflicted injury that is not consistent with a clotting disorder, vasculitis, reasonable cultural practices, or other nonintentional injury circumstances.

Recommended Reading

Buchwald D, Panwala S, Hooton TM. Use of traditional health practices by Southeast Asian refugees in a primary care clinic. *West J Med.* 1992;156:507–511

Chapter 17

Fever and Rash for 3 Days

Presentation

A 21-month-old previously healthy boy arrives in the emergency department (ED) on day 3 of a febrile illness. On the first day of fever, he developed a rash that affected his face first, then spread throughout his body. The following day, his lips became redder. Today, his palms and soles are reddened. Although he vomited on the first day of the illness, he has had no other gastrointestinal or respiratory symptoms. He has been irritable and crying, although the exact source of discomfort is unclear. He has been taking fluids poorly and is unwilling to stand or walk. His parents have been administering acetaminophen and ibuprofen, which they started only after the onset of the rash.

Examination reveals fever (temperature 38.6°C) and tachycardia (184 beats/min) but normal blood pressure (96/64), good perfusion, and unlabored respirations. Although irritable, he is alert and consolable by his mother, with whom he interacts in an otherwise age-appropriate manner. Conjunctivae are not injected. His lips are reddened and mildly cracked, with prominent lingual papillae laterally (Figure 17-1). His oropharynx is otherwise normal and there is no tonsillar exudate. Cardiac and respiratory examinations are normal. He has no splenomegaly or adenopathy. Palmar and plantar surfaces are diffusely erythematous (Figure 17-2). An erythematous macular exanthema covers the extremities and nearly becomes confluent on the trunk. The scrotum is diffusely erythematous with scaling (Figure 17-3). Extremity tenderness and joint effusions are absent.

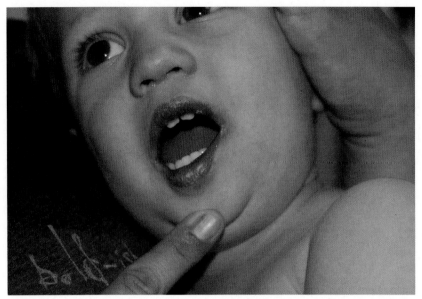

Figure 17-1

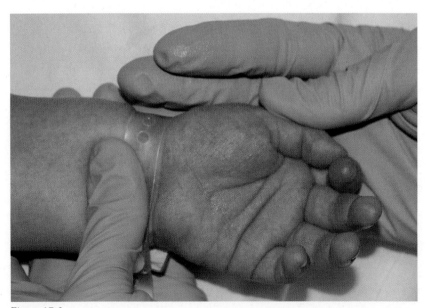

Figure 17-2

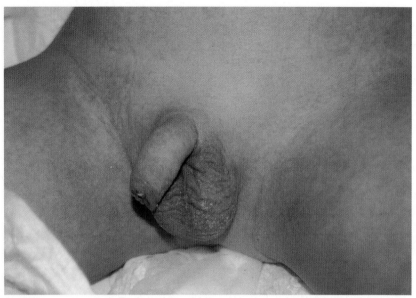

Figure 17-3

Discussion

Differential Diagnosis
- Viral exanthem
- Drug reaction
- Staphylococcal scalded skin syndrome
- Scarlet fever
- Kawasaki disease (KD)
- Toxic shock syndrome
- Stevens-Johnson syndrome

Evaluation
The absence of skin separation makes staphylococcal scalded skin syndrome, Stevens-Johnson syndrome, and toxic epidermal necrolysis unlikely. Streptococcal scarlet fever is uncommon in this age group, and the patient lacks an exudative pharyngitis. Toxic shock (staphylococcal or streptococcal) might have similar mucocutaneous manifestations, but your patient is normotensive. This patient presents with fewer days of fever and with fewer criteria

(3 of 5 clinical criteria) than traditionally required for the clinical diagnosis of KD (Box 17-1). He has a generalized rash, palmar and plantar erythema, and a strawberry tongue with red, cracked lips. He lacks cervical adenopathy and conjunctival injection. Although the scrotal and perineal component of the rash and the history of limb pain are highly suggestive, they are not among the criteria. Nonetheless, this ED visit represents an opportunity to make an early diagnosis. Laboratory studies include white blood cells (WBC) 7,100/µL with 22% band forms, erythrocyte sedimentation rate 66 mm/h, C-reactive protein 11.9 mg/dL, gamma glutamyl transpeptidase 75 U/L, alanine aminotransferase 232 U/L, aspartate aminotransferase 245 U/L, and urine obtained by bag contains 10 to 20 WBC/high-power field.

Box 17-1. Diagnostic Criteria for Kawasaki Disease

Fever of at least 5 days' duration,[a] plus at least 4 of the following[b]:

Extremity changes
    Acute: Palmar, plantar erythema; hand, foot swelling
    Subacute: Desquamation of fingers and toes in a periungual distribution
    (week 2–3 of illness)

Polymorphous exanthem
Bilateral conjunctival injection without exudates
Oral changes (cracked, red lips; strawberry tongue; mucosal injection)
Cervical adenopathy >1.5 cm
Exclusion of other diseases

[a] By convention, each calendar day is included as a day of illness. Diagnosis is possible on day 4 when at least 4 criteria are present. Experienced clinicians may make the diagnosis before day 4.
[b] In the presence of coronary artery abnormalities, the diagnosis may be made with less than 4 criteria.
Adapted from Newburger JW, Takahashi M, Gerber MA, et al. Diagnosis, treatment, and long-term management of Kawasaki disease: a statement for health professionals from the Committee on Rheumatic Fever, Endocarditis, and Kawasaki disease, Council on Cardiovascular Disease in the Young, American Heart Association. *Pediatrics*. 2004;114:1708–1733

Treatment

The striking evidence of inflammation and other laboratory abnormalities are impossible to ignore. Kawasaki disease becomes the leading diagnosis, which leads to admission for treatment with intravenous immunoglobulin (IVIG) (2 g/kg) and high-dose aspirin. Although this patient briefly improves, his fever recurs, and he receives a second infusion of IVIG before discharge. His echocardiogram reveals no coronary artery abnormalities.

Keep in Mind

Although KD is most common in Japan and among children of Japanese ancestry, all racial groups are affected. The traditional diagnostic criteria ($\geq$5 days of fever and $\geq$4 of 5 clinical features) were originally designed for epidemiologic surveillance. They lack sufficient sensitivity in individual patients and do not allow for the diagnosis of early or incomplete KD. Prompt diagnosis is important because coronary artery lesions develop in 20% to 25% of patients not treated within the first 10 days of illness, including those with incomplete KD. Damage to the coronary arteries can be detected as early as the second or third day of fever. On the other hand, injudicious use of IVIG for illnesses that vaguely resemble KD incurs the cost of hospital admission and medication administration as well as risks of hypotension, wheezing, serum sickness, renal failure, and bloodborne disease transmission.

In the absence of a specific diagnostic test, the diagnosis rests on a combination of clinical evaluation and nonspecific screening tests. The American Heart Association guidelines include an algorithm that allows for the diagnosis of KD on the fourth day of fever with 4 of 5 clinical criteria and on the fifth day (or later) of fever with less than 4 criteria but are silent on the combination of short duration and insufficient number of clinical criteria. These guidelines do not specifically dictate diagnosis and treatment at 3 days of illness. However, the guidelines state that clinicians with significant experience in treating KD may make the diagnosis before day 4 of fever to facilitate more accurate and timely diagnosis. Therefore, clinicians who doubt the diagnosis of KD and opt for outpatient observation must weigh the benefit of increased diagnostic accuracy with deferred diagnosis and treatment against the risk of delayed treatment or nontreatment if the patient fails to comply with outpatient follow-up.

When a child with suspected KD presents with more than 5 days of fever and with classic clinical findings, the diagnosis and decision to admit are not in question. The clinical challenge lies in the recognition of KD in patients with early presentations or incomplete or atypical clinical manifestations. Incomplete presentations are more common among infants younger than 6 months, and infants younger than 12 months are also at greater risk of coronary artery abnormalities. Ongoing research is likely to result in continued modification of the diagnostic criteria and more specific laboratory markers for KD. Future work may also shed light on the role and utility of aspirin therapy and on the use of newer antiinflammatory therapies such as tumor necrosis factor antagonists in IVIG failure.

Recommended Reading

American Academy of Pediatrics. Kawasaki disease. In: Pickering LK, Baker CJ, Kimberlin DW, Long SS, eds. *Red Book: 2009 Report of the Committee on Infectious Diseases*. 28th ed. Elk Grove Village, IL: American Academy of Pediatrics; 2009:413–418

Newburger JW, Takahashi M, Gerber MA, et al. Diagnosis, treatment, and long-term management of Kawasaki disease: a statement for health professionals from the Committee on Rheumatic Fever, Endocarditis, and Kawasaki disease, Council on Cardiovascular Disease in the Young, American Heart Association. *Pediatrics*. 2004;114:1708–1733

Chapter 18

Amoxicillin and Ibuprofen Allergy

Presentation

A 3-year-old girl has a history of fever since yesterday. Her temperature has been measured as high as 39.4°C. She has mild nasal congestion and a mild cough. Her oral intake is reduced, but her fluid intake and urine output are good. There is no vomiting or diarrhea. Her parents gave her acetaminophen, which lowered her temperature. However, the fever returned approximately 3 hours later, so her parents decided to bring her to the emergency department (ED).

Past medical history is unremarkable except for penicillin allergy. There is no history of prematurity, urinary tract infection, or pneumonia.

Social history is negative. However, family history reveals that 2 cousins have colds. The child's immunizations are up to date.

Examination reveals the following vital signs: tympanic temperature 38.3°C, pulse 90 beats/min, respiration 30 breaths/min, and blood pressure 85/50 mm Hg. She is alert, active, and cooperative, and she is not toxic or irritable. Her eyes and tympanic membranes are normal. Her nose is clear at this time. Her pharynx reveals tonsillar exudates. Her mucosa is moist. Her neck is supple with small, palpable nodes. Heart, lungs, and abdomen are normal. Color and perfusion are good.

Discussion

Differential Diagnosis
- Fever
- Exudative tonsillitis
- Streptococcal tonsillitis
- Viral tonsillitis

Evaluation
Because of the persistent fever, a dose of ibuprofen is provided, and a rapid streptococcal antigen swab of her throat is ordered. An urticarial rash is noted 20 minutes later—an allergic reaction to the ibuprofen. No wheezing or lip swelling is present.

The rapid streptococcal antigen study returns positive. A presumptive diagnosis of streptococcal tonsillitis is made. Unfortunately, the patient has a history of penicillin allergy, so more history is obtained.

Treatment
She is administered a dose of oral diphenhydramine, and the rash resolves within 30 minutes.

Keep in Mind
Commonly asked questions about drug allergies that are potentially useful include the following: What happens when the drug is taken? How was the drug administered? What similar drugs can the patient take?

What happens when she takes penicillin? In some instances, the answer is often a known side effect of the drug rather than an allergic reaction. For example, when diarrhea results from amoxicillin, this is most often an adverse effect of the drug rather than an allergic reaction. A rash reaction to amoxicillin could suggest that this is an allergic reaction. An urticarial rash is more likely to be a hypersensitivity (allergic) mechanism, but many nonurticarial rashes could be the result of nonallergic etiologies—the so-called amoxicillin rash that occurs when a particular virus and amoxicillin combine to result in a nonallergic rash similar to the rash that results from infectious mononucleosis and ampicillin. This means that if amoxicillin is given in the future, such a rash would not result. A more serious reaction characterized by, for example, passing out, pallor, wheezing, or airway swelling suggests that the allergy is severe.

How was the penicillin administered? Long-acting intramuscular (IM) penicillin injections are less commonly administered in recent years than in previous decades (so this could apply to teens and adults). Patients who received long-acting (benzathine or procaine) penicillin IM injections may have been reacting to unintentional intravenous (IV) injections of crystalline penicillin, rather than experiencing a true allergic reaction. These penicillin injection preparations are white and opaque, which renders the standard method of avoiding an intravascular injection ineffective. Drawing back on the syringe plunger before the injection to see whether a flash of blood enters the syringe is the standard method, but if the needle tip is in a vein, the blood would enter the central portion of the syringe barrel, which would not be visible in the outer syringe barrel because the crystalline penicillin is opaque.

Further, long-acting penicillins contain other drugs such as procaine and benzathine. The patient could potentially be allergic to these substances instead of the penicillin. Intramuscular ceftriaxone is frequently administered in EDs, clinics, and primary care offices. Some clinicians prefer to dilute the ceftriaxone with lidocaine instead of sterile water or saline to reduce the pain of the ceftriaxone injection. However, if an allergic reaction results, it is unclear whether the patient is reacting to ceftriaxone or lidocaine. Patients are often not told about the lidocaine, so patients conclude that they are allergic to ceftriaxone.

What other antibiotics can she take? This question is particularly useful because it helps confirm which antibiotics are likely to be safe. In some instances, the allergy is actually removed from consideration. For example, a parent might say that her child is allergic to amoxicillin but that the child has subsequently taken amoxicillin-clavulanate, which essentially rules out amoxicillin allergy. Someone prescribed the amoxicillin-clavulanate in error to an amoxicillin-allergic patient, but this history is fairly common. A history of taking cephalosporins without any problems is also useful because some penicillin-allergic patients are also allergic to cephalosporins.

Group A streptococci are still sensitive to penicillin and cephalosporins.
Once the allergy history is clarified, most penicillin-allergic patients can
be treated with cephalosporins. Other treatment possibilities include
erythromycin or clindamycin. Some group A streptococci are resistant
to erythromycin and clindamycin, but antibiotic sensitivity patters are
subject to change.

Of particular importance is that this patient had a witnessed allergic reaction to ibuprofen. Most patients who are allergic to ibuprofen are also
allergic to salicylates. Unlike antibiotics, salicylates and related products
are available over the counter. Therefore, patients must be told what to
avoid. Patients who are allergic to ibuprofen should be told to avoid all
salicylates and nonsteroidal antiinflammatory drugs, which include the
drugs listed in Box 18-1.

Box 18-1. Nonsteroidal Antiinflammatory Drugs

Naproxen
Aspirin
Ibuprofen
Anacin, Excedrin, Bufferin, Bayer (Various contain combinations of aspirin, ibuprofen, and/or acetaminophen.)
Dysmenorrhea medications such as Midol (usually contain ibuprofen)
Aspercreme (trolamine salicylate)[a]
Many other topical pain rubs (eg, Icy Hot, Salonpas, some Bengay products [methyl salicylate])
Pepto-Bismol (bismuth subsalicylate)
Combination cold remedies (Many of these contain ibuprofen.)

[a]This product specifically states that it does not contain aspirin.

Recommended Reading

Salkind AR, Cuddy PG, Foxworth JW. The rational clinical examination.
    Is this patient allergic to penicillin? An evidence-based analysis of the
    likelihood of penicillin allergy. *JAMA.* 2001;285:2498–2505

Chapter 19

Fever, Vomiting, Diarrhea, and Rash

Presentation

A 7-year-old boy developed fever 4 days ago, along with vomiting, diarrhea, and headache, as well as anorexia for solid food. He also had a sore throat, rhinorrhea, and a cough, which worsened in the latter days of the illness. Last night, a rash appeared over his arms and legs, and his eyes became red with a scant discharge. He has no ill contacts. The only treatment consists of antipyretics. Nine days previously, he saw his pediatrician for a purulent conjunctivitis and received a prescription for a fluoroquinolone ophthalmic solution. He has a long-standing history of asthma, for which he infrequently uses an albuterol metered dose inhaler.

He is mildly febrile (38.3°C) and tachycardic (112 beats/min) with otherwise normal vital signs and perfusion. His conjunctivae are injected bilaterally (Figure 19-1), without clear limbal sparing or exudate. A clear nasal discharge is present. He has a mildly exudative pharyngitis, and the rest of his mucous membranes appear somewhat erythematous. His lips are cracked and blistered. He has 1- to 1.5-cm cervical lymph nodes bilaterally. His abdomen is mildly tender without localization. Extremities are well perfused and demonstrate no joint swelling or arthralgias. A diffuse blanching erythematous macular rash covers his face, trunk, and extremities. You note a subtle target-shaped configuration to some of the lesions. Many of the lesions are coalescent, especially on his arms (Figure 19-2). There is mild extension of the eruption to his genitalia. No blistering or other epidermal loss is evident.

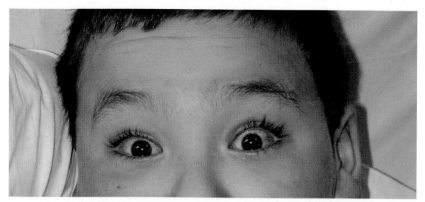

Figure 19-1

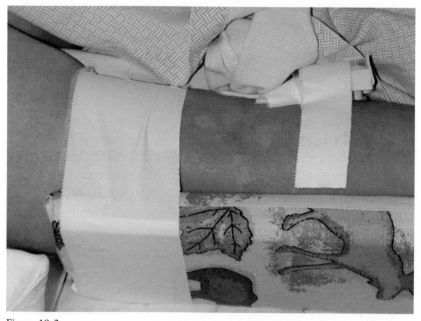

Figure 19-2

Discussion

Differential Diagnosis

- Scarlet fever
- Stevens-Johnson syndrome
- Toxic epidermal necrolysis
- Drug reaction
- Viral infection
- Kawasaki disease (KD)
- Toxic shock syndrome

Evaluation

The entities with the most serious consequences and most effective specific therapies are Stevens-Johnson syndrome or toxic epidermal necrolysis, and KD. The benign hemodynamic status makes toxic shock syndrome unlikely. The other diagnoses are more likely to benefit from supportive care. The patient is, therefore, admitted for observation, consultation, and supportive care. Nonsteroidal antiinflammatory medications are withheld because they are a possible precipitating agent for Stevens-Johnson syndrome.

Initial laboratory evaluation includes the following results: white blood cell (WBC) count 12,200/µL (60% neutrophils, 16% band forms, 18% lymphocytes, and 6% monocytes), erythrocyte sedimentation rate (ESR) 32 mm/h, hemoglobin 13.6 g/dL, platelets 320,000/µL, C-reactive protein (CRP) 7.1 mg/dL, alanine aminotransferase (ALT) 24 U/L, and urine 5 WBC per high-power field. The result from a streptococcal antigen test of a throat swab is negative.

Treatment

During hospital observation, no epidermal loss is noted. An increase in temperature to 39.2°C occurs during the first 2 hospital days. The impression of the consulting ophthalmologist is of KD or a viral illness. The boy develops a white strawberry tongue (Figure 19-3) and hand and foot swelling (Figure 19-4), which prompt further concern for evolving KD. However, copious nasal discharge is also present. C-reactive protein levels remain high (6.8 mg/dL), but there are no worrisome changes in WBC (9,800/µL), platelet count (293,000/µL), ESR (35 mm/h), or gamma glutamyl transferase

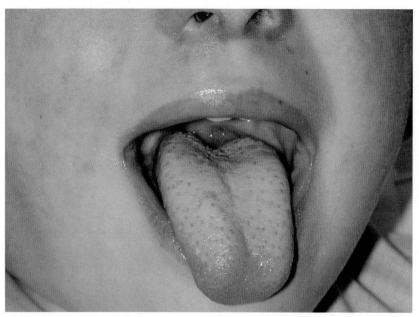

Figure 19-3

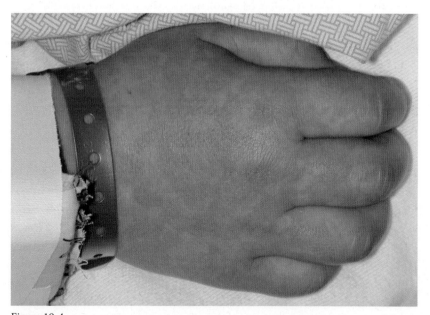

Figure 19-4

(GGT) (22 U/L). Serologic tests reveal evidence of previous Epstein-Barr virus infection but no evidence of acute mycoplasma infection. By the morning of the third hospital day, the patient still has a fever (38.7°C), but an immunofluorescent antigen test of nasopharyngeal scrapings is positive for the detection of adenovirus. The patient is discharged with instructions for symptom relief and recovers uneventfully.

Keep in Mind

Adenoviral infection is extremely common in infancy and early childhood, and it has a wide range of clinical manifestations. Adenoviruses account for up to 24% of childhood respiratory illnesses, including nasopharyngitis, pharyngoconjunctival fever, croup, bronchiolitis, and pneumonia (which may occasionally be severe and even fatal). Adenoviruses also account for 5% to 15% of childhood diarrheal illness and have been implicated in hepatitis, mesenteric adenitis, and intussusception. Other localized manifestations include epidemic keratoconjunctivitis and hemorrhagic cystitis. Viremia gives rise to systemic manifestations as well as exanthema (most commonly maculopapular but also morbilliform or petechial), which may cause confusion with KD.

The manifestations of KD are similar to those of streptococcal infection, Epstein-Barr infection, measles, other viral infections, drug reactions, and rheumatologic diseases. Among mimickers of KD, adenoviral infection is most likely to cause difficulty in differentiation because of the overlap of clinical features and the lack of widespread availability of a rapid pathogen-specific diagnostic test. Features more likely to be present in KD include conjunctival changes, extremity changes, and perineal accentuation of the exanthem. Adenoviral disease more often has a purulent conjunctivitis and an exudative pharyngitis. Although KD more often has abnormalities of WBC, ESR, CRP, ALT, albumin, and GGT, adenoviral infection may manifest with impressive laboratory evidence of inflammation. When present, pyuria and anterior uveitis help differentiate KD from adenoviral infection.

When the diagnosis of a febrile exanthem is in doubt but includes potential serious illness, observation (either inpatient or outpatient) without treatment may be useful. When an illness has some features consistent with KD along with atypical features (such as prominent respiratory symptoms, as in this case), a positive adenoviral antigen detection test may obviate the need for a more extensive evaluation and the costs and risks of intravenous immunoglobulin therapy.

Recommended Reading

Barone SR, Pontrelli LR, Krilov LR. The differentiation of classic Kawasaki disease, atypical Kawasaki disease, and acute adenoviral infection: use of clinical features and a rapid direct fluorescent antigen test. *Arch Pediatr Adolesc Med.* 2000;154:453–456

Cherry JD. Adenoviruses. In: Feigin RD, Cherry JD, Demmler GJ, Kaplan SL, eds. *Textbook of Pediatric Infectious Diseases.* 5th ed. Philadelphia, PA: WB Saunders; 2004:1843–1863

Chapter 20

Extremity Peeling After Febrile Illness

Presentation

A 7-month-old girl presents to your emergency department (ED) on day 4 of a febrile illness with temperatures up to 39.5°C. A truncal and perineal rash developed from day 2, as did redness and cracking of the lips and mild conjunctival injection. No hand and foot changes have occurred other than extension of the truncal rash. There have been cough, rhinorrhea, and diarrhea with no vomiting. Parents report no neck swelling and no apparent limb pain. Her primary physician reports her to be irritable. Before this illness, she was completely healthy, took no medications, and was fully vaccinated.

Laboratory tests obtained the day before reveal the following: normal white blood cell (WBC) count of 10,600/μL with unremarkable differential, hemoglobin 10.5 g/dL, and platelets 295,000/μL. She is afebrile (37.1°C) but has just received acetaminophen. Although she is tachycardic (172 beats/min) while crying, she appears otherwise well perfused and calm in her mother's arms. She has mild conjunctival injection, and her lips are cracked and reddened. There are no lingual changes or cervical adenopathy. A scant nasal discharge is present. There is no adenopathy other than shotty inguinal nodes. A sparse macular exanthem covers the trunk and extremities with diffuse erythema over the labia majora. The hands and feet are neither swollen nor red. No joint effusion is present.

Discussion

Differential Diagnosis

- Kawasaki disease (KD)
- Viral infection with exanthem
- Scarlet fever (unusual in this age group)
- Staphylococcal scalded skin syndrome
- Drug reaction

Evaluation

Screening laboratory test results include the following: WBC 10,300/μL with normal differential count, hemoglobin 10.7 g/dL, platelets 287,000/μL, erythrocyte sedimentation rate (ESR) 22 mm/h, and normal values for transaminases, albumin, and gamma glutamyl transpeptidase. The sole abnormalities are a C-reactive protein (CRP) of 5.8 mg/dL and urine (obtained by bag) that contains 10 to 20 WBC/hpf. The symptoms and laboratory results suggest a mildly prolonged infectious illness, likely of viral origin, but do not exclude KD. However, because the patient meets only 3 of the 5 clinical criteria for KD and because she presents sufficiently early to begin intravenous immunoglobulin (IVIG) if the illness progresses in the next several days, an outpatient observation plan is developed. Discharge teaching includes symptomatic care measures, direction to follow up with the primary care physician in 1 or 2 days, and instructions to return if the child gets worse or new concerns appear.

While at home, the patient continues to be somewhat more irritable than usual. Since her first ED visit, she has no longer had measured fevers, but her parents continue to periodically administer acetaminophen. The patient does not arrive for follow-up with her usual primary physician until 14 days later, by which time she has developed peeling skin on her fingertips and toes. She has residual cough and rhinorrhea but continues to behave normally and eat well. She is again directed to the ED, where the results of her physical examination are normal other than desquamation of the fingers and toes in a periungual distribution (figures 20-1 to 20-4). Her hands and feet have no erythema, edema, or apparent tenderness to palpation.

Repeat laboratory results include the following findings: WBC 10,100/μL, hemoglobin 11.1 g/dL, platelets 525,000/μL, ESR 64 mm/h, and CRP less than 0.3 mg/dL.

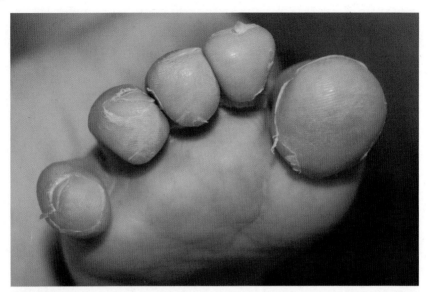

Figure 20-1

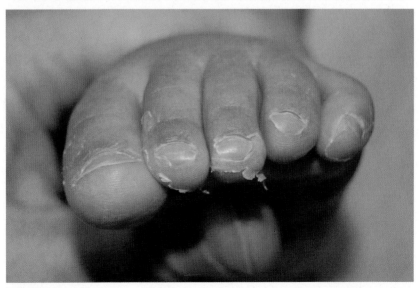

Figure 20-2

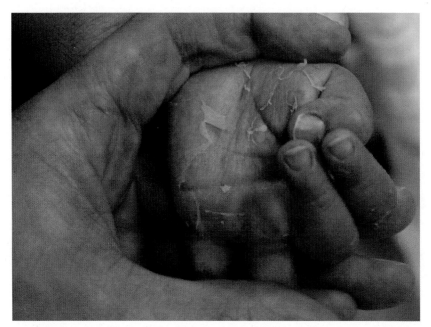

Figure 20-3

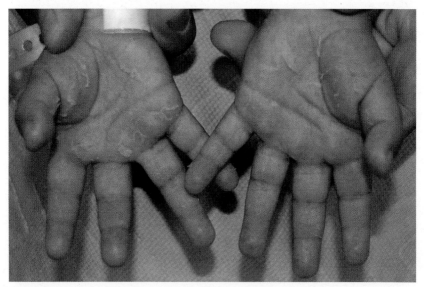

Figure 20-4

Treatment

The periungual peeling constitutes a fourth clinical criterion for KD, and the elevated ESR reflects persistent inflammation even in the absence of fever. You admit the patient for further evaluation and treatment. An echocardiogram performed after admission reveals normal coronary arteries but does not exclude the diagnosis of KD. The patient receives IVIG 2 g/kg and because she is now afebrile and has no coronary artery lesions, low-dose aspirin.

Keep in Mind

Kawasaki disease is a febrile vasculitis whose diagnosis primarily depends on clinical criteria as well as suggestive but nonspecific laboratory abnormalities. Treatment with IVIG by day 10 of illness is known to reduce the risk of coronary artery abnormalities. However, in the absence of a specific test, a conclusive or timely diagnosis is sometimes hard to make. Estimates of rates of late diagnosis (after 10 days of illness) range from 16% to 28%. The delay to diagnosis usually depends on the time required for clinicians to arrive at the diagnosis rather than parental health care–seeking behavior. Patients at risk for late diagnosis are younger than 6 months, have incomplete clinical criteria, and have clinical findings that appear over a longer period. A unique phenomenon occurs along the United States-Mexico border; seeking health care in Mexico appears to be a risk factor for the delayed diagnosis of KD, possibly due to the fragmentation of medical care on return to the United States. Because the clinical criteria need not be present concurrently, the clinician must carefully seek a history of physical findings compatible with KD that may have resolved before the patient sought care. When the constellation of findings is incomplete but suggests KD, the clinician should obtain laboratory tests of inflammation (especially CBC, ESR, and CRP). If an equivocal picture persists, an echocardiogram is warranted. If the diagnosis or appropriate treatment course is uncertain, expert consultation should be considered.

The patient in this case sought care on day 4 of fever with only 3 of the principal criteria of KD and only 1 abnormal laboratory value. In the otherwise well-appearing patient, this early presentation represented an opportunity to monitor the patient closely on an outpatient basis with repeated laboratory tests as dictated by the clinical course. Counseling parents about the clinical signs of KD and the significance of periungual desquamation in the convalescent phase can help to ensure that patients return for evaluation should these signs appear. In this situation, the patient did not seek follow-up care until peeling occurred. Echocardiography is the next step. However, even when the diagnosis occurs after day 10 of illness, treatment with IVIG is warranted when fever or increased levels of inflammatory markers reflect persistent inflammation.

Recommended Reading

American Academy of Pediatrics. Kawasaki disease. In: Pickering LK, Baker CJ, Kimberlin DW, Long SS, eds. *Red Book: 2009 Report of the Committee on Infectious Diseases.* 28th ed. Elk Grove Village, IL: American Academy of Pediatrics: 2009:413–418

Anderson MS, Todd JK, Glodé MP. Delayed diagnosis of Kawasaki syndrome: an analysis of the problem. *Pediatrics.* 2005;115:e428–e433

Minich LL, Sleeper LA, Atz AM, et al. Delayed diagnosis of Kawasaki disease: what are the risk factors? *Pediatrics.* 2007;120:e1434–e1440

Newburger JW, Takahashi M, Gerber MA, et al. Diagnosis, treatment, and long-term management of Kawasaki disease: a statement for health professionals from the Committee on Rheumatic Fever, Endocarditis, and Kawasaki disease, Council on Cardiovascular Disease in the Young, American Heart Association. *Pediatrics.* 2004;114:1708–1733

Wilder MS, Palinkas LA, Kao AS, Bastian JF, Turner CL, Burns JC. Delayed diagnosis by physicians contributes to the development of coronary artery aneurysms in children with Kawasaki syndrome. *Pediatr Infect Dis J.* 2007;26:256–260

Chapter 21

Rash and Blistering With Fever for 2 Days

Presentation

A previously healthy 5-year-old girl arrives in the emergency department (ED) with a 2-day history of fever and a rash with blistering. The illness began with diarrhea, which resolved. The patient developed a low-grade fever (38°C) that increased to 40°C during evaluation at an outside clinic. The rash began with facial erythema and swollen eyelids. It became a pruritic rash and spread over the trunk, arms, and perineum with cutaneous and intraoral vesication. The patient has had a productive cough and rhinorrhea. She has been eating and drinking less, but her parents report normal urine output and stools and she has not been vomiting. Her family reports no allergies to medications, foods, or environmental allergens, and her only medications have been acetaminophen and diphenhydramine, both of which were begun after the onset of fever and rash.

She underwent evaluation at another hospital yesterday. Available results include the following laboratory values: white blood cell (WBC) count 5,200/μL, platelets 178,000/μL, sodium 135 mmol/L, potassium 3.4 mmol/L, glucose 132 mg/dL, alkaline phosphatase 149 U/L, aspartate aminotransferase (AST) 138 U/L, alanine aminotransferase (ALT) 91 U/L, and urinalysis positive for moderate hematuria and ketonuria.

Now in the ED, she is febrile (temperature 38.4°C) and tachycardic (137 beats/min), but alert and well perfused with normal blood pressure (106/67 mm Hg) and in no respiratory distress. Her eyelids are edematous and erythematous with bilateral conjunctival injection and exudate (Figure 21-1). Her lips are reddened with regions of cracking and denuding, and the tongue shows early desquamation on the lateral surfaces (Figure 21-2). Flaccid blisters cover both cheeks and the chin (figures 21-3 and 21-4). Erythematous macules cover the palms, and the fingertips are diffusely erythematous (Figure 21-5). The torso has a diffuse macular eruption with scattered regions of vesication and desquamation (Figure 21-6). The rash extends into the perineum. Examination of heart, lungs, and extremities is normal. No lymphadenopathy or hepatosplenomegaly is present.

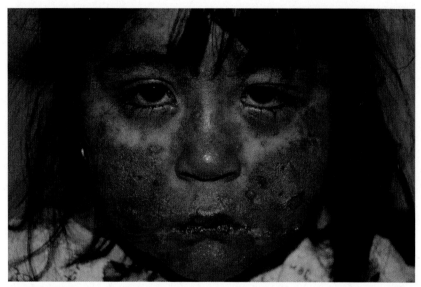

Figure 21-1

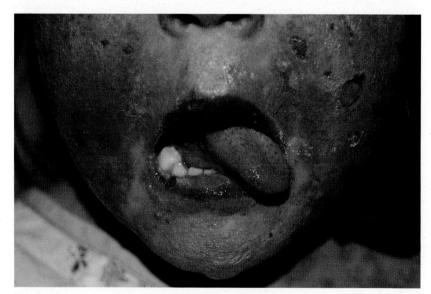

Figure 21-2

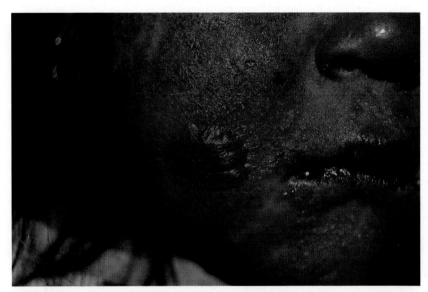

Figure 21-3

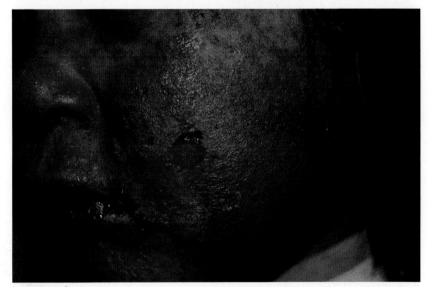

Figure 21-4

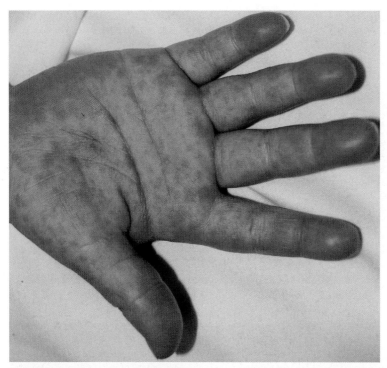

Figure 21-5

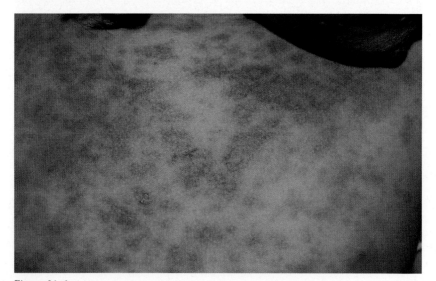

Figure 21-6

Discussion

Differential Diagnosis

- Stevens-Johnson syndrome (SJS)
- Toxic epidermal necrolysis (TEN)
- Thermal or chemical injury
- Staphylococcal scalded skin syndrome
- Kawasaki disease
- Erythema multiforme

Evaluation

The results of laboratory studies are as follows: erythrocyte sedimentation rate 20 mm/h, C-reactive protein 5.2 mg/dL, WBC 4,900/μL, hemoglobin 12.2 g/dL, platelet count 73,000/μL, gamma glutamyl transpeptidase 445 U/L, AST 129 U/L, and ALT 92 U/L. Electrolytes are normal. Urinalysis reveals 1+ ketonuria and 8 to 10 WBC/high-power field (hpf) and 10 to 12 red blood cells/hpf.

Treatment

On the basis of initial clinical evaluation and laboratory abnormalities, this patient likely has SJS. She is admitted to the hospital for treatment and monitoring. Along with dermatology and ophthalmology consultations, she receives a 4-day course of intravenous immunoglobulin (IVIG) 1 g/kg per day. Local wound care consists of gentle cleansing, antibiotic ointment, and nonadherent dressings until her skin has healed. By the fourth hospital day, skin involvement increases to more than 30%, warranting a diagnosis of TEN.

She receives a 5-day course of azithromycin because of serologic evidence of mycoplasma infection. Respiratory distress and hypoxia develop, which are attributed to involvement of respiratory epithelium and require a 3-week period of endotracheal intubation and mechanical ventilation. Electrolyte balance and renal function remain normal. Eye care consists of topical corticosteroid, antibiotic, and cycloplegic drops until her condition begins to improve. After epithelial healing is well established, she is discharged home with prescriptions for artificial tears and emollients.

Keep in Mind

Stevens-Johnson syndrome and TEN are uncommon skin eruptions that are associated with substantial morbidity and mortality. Fever, epidermal detachment (characteristically flaccid blisters), and mucositis are common, but substantial ocular, gastrointestinal, and respiratory sequelae also occur. Medications trigger most cases, with antibiotics (particularly sulfonamides), anticonvulsants (phenobarbital, phenytoin, and carbamazepine), and non-steroidal antiinflammatory drugs implicated most frequently. Mycoplasma and other infectious agents may also trigger SJS and TEN.

Skin loss occurs at the level of the dermal-epidermal junction and is consequently more severe than that associated with staphylococcal scalded skin syndrome, which involves an intraepidermal cleavage plane. The extent of epidermal loss determines the diagnostic category as well as prognosis. Stevens-Johnson syndrome involves less than 10% of body surface area and has a 1% to 5% mortality. Toxic epidermal necrolysis is present when epidermal loss is greater than 30% and has a mortality rate of approximately 30%. Epidermal loss of 10% to 30% of the body surface area defines the SJS-TEN overlap. Prompt discontinuation of the offending agent and initiation of aggressive supportive care in a critical care or burn unit setting are crucial. Intravenous immunoglobulin in total doses greater than 2 g/kg appears to result in a decrease in mortality in TEN. In SJS, IVIG halts disease progression and decreases time to complete healing.

Recommended Reading

French LE. Toxic epidermal necrolysis and Stevens-Johnson syndrome: our current understanding. *Allergol Int.* 2006;55:9–16

Metry DW, Jung P, Levy ML. Use of intravenous immunoglobulin in children with Stevens-Johnson syndrome and toxic epidermal necrolysis: seven cases and review of the literature. *Pediatrics.* 2003;112:1430–1436

Paller AS, Mancini AJ. The hypersensitivity syndromes. In: Paller AS, Mancini AJ. *Hurwitz Clinical Pediatric Dermatology: A Textbook of Skin Disorders of Childhood and Adolescence.* 3rd ed. Philadelphia, PA: WB Saunders; 2005:525–556

Pereira FA, Mudgil AV, Rosmarin DM. Toxic epidermal necrolysis. *J Am Acad Dermatol.* 2007;56:181–200

Chapter 22

Fever and Facial Puffiness

Presentation

A 3-year-old girl arrives at the emergency department (ED) with fever and facial swelling. Fever was noted earlier today. Her mother measured the temperature at 39.5°C. Acetaminophen was provided and the child defervesced, but fever returned 3 hours later. There is no runny nose, coughing, vomiting, or diarrhea. The facial swelling was noticed 5 weeks ago. She went to her primary care physician, who ordered some blood tests. They tried to obtain a urine sample that day, but she was not willing or able to void. Her mother was told that the blood tests were normal. Because everything was normal, there was not much to do. She did not return to her primary care physician because the facial swelling would periodically improve. Her urine output is less than it normally is.

Past medical history is negative; family and social history are not contributory.

Examination reveals the following vital signs: oral temperature 38.7°C, pulse 95 beats/min, respiration 25 breaths/min, blood pressure 85/55 mm Hg, and oxygen saturation 99% in room air. Her face is visibly edematous. She is alert, subdued, and cooperative. Her conjunctiva is clear. There is obvious periorbital edema. Tympanic membranes, nose, and mouth are normal. Neck is supple without adenopathy. Heart and lungs are normal. Her abdomen is soft and mildly tender with possible ascites. Bowel sounds are normoactive. There are no inguinal hernias. Mild labial edema is present. Her overall color is slightly pale. There is mild pitting edema over her tibiae.

Discussion

Differential Diagnosis
- Fever
- Viral infection
- Nephrotic syndrome
- Pneumococcal sepsis

Evaluation
A complete blood count was ordered with the following findings: white blood cells 28,000/μL, 32% segmented neutrophils, 33% bands, 5% metamyelocytes, 30% lymphocytes, hemoglobin 13 g/dL, hematocrit 39%, and platelet count 110,000/μL. Results of a blood culture are pending. Chemistry results are as follows: sodium 136 mmol/L, potassium 4.0 mmol/L, chloride 100 mmol/L, and bicarbonate 19 mmol/L. Her creatinine is 0.3 mg/dL and her blood urea nitrogen is 8 mg/dL. Albumin is 2.9 g/dL and total protein is 4.9 g/dL. Liver enzymes are normal. Urinalysis reveals 3 to 5 red blood cells per high-power field and 4+ protein, but otherwise, everything is normal.

Treatment
Cefotaxime and vancomycin are administered. Blood cultures yielded growth of *Streptococcus pneumoniae* and the patient recovered without sequelae.

Keep in Mind

This patient's proteinuria and hypoalbuminemia suffice to make the ED diagnosis of nephrotic syndrome. If serum cholesterol and lipids were ordered, these values should be high in most patients with nephrosis. The most common cause of childhood nephrosis is minimal change disease sometimes called lipoid nephrosis, nil disease, or idiopathic childhood nephrosis. Minimal change disease typically improves with a course of corticosteroids.

The fever and leukocytosis indicate the possibility of sepsis. Patients with nephrotic syndrome are more susceptible to pneumococcal sepsis. Most pneumococci are sensitive to penicillin. However, intermediate penicillin resistance has emerged. This can be overcome by increasing the doses of penicillins and cephalosporins to overwhelm the penicillin-binding proteins. High-level pneumococcal resistance has also emerged, requiring vancomycin therapy.

Immunocompromised patients are at higher risk of sepsis. Such patients should not be assumed to have viral infections as the cause of their fever. Patients without spleens are at high risk for sepsis. A left upper quadrant scar suggests the possibility that the spleen has been surgically removed. Patients with a history of serious abdominal trauma or chronic idiopathic thrombocytopenic purpura might have been treated with a splenectomy. Patients with sickle cell anemia have functional asplenia because their spleen slowly undergoes infarction. Cancer and leukemia patients undergoing chemotherapy and children with known immunodeficiency conditions are at high risk of sepsis. Broad-spectrum antibiotics that include *Pseudomonas* coverage should be empirically initiated for such patients.

Recommended Reading

Cronan KM, Kost SI. Renal and electrolyte emergencies. In: Fleisher GR, Ludwig S, Henretig FM, Ruddy RM, Silverman BK, eds. *Textbook of Pediatric Emergency Medicine.* 5th ed. Philadelphia, PA: Lippincott Williams & Wilkins; 2006:873–919

Chapter 23

Fever and Hives

Presentation

A 3-year-old African American girl is brought into the emergency department (ED) with fever and hives. Her mother treated her with acetaminophen and diphenhydramine. These medications helped the fever but did
not change the rash, which seems to be itchy. Her highest temperature at
home was 38.4°C. She has a mild cough and says that her throat hurts. There
is no vomiting or diarrhea. Her appetite is reduced, but she is drinking and
urinating well. There are no known ill contacts, but she goes to preschool.

Past medical history is negative.

Examination reveals the following vital signs: oral temperature 38.4°C,
pulse 125 beats/min, respiration 26 breaths/min, blood pressure 85/55 mm
Hg, and oxygen saturation 99% in room air. She is alert and cooperative,
in no distress. No conjunctival injection is noted. Tympanic membranes
are normal. Her pharynx appears normal. Tonsils are not enlarged. Her
tongue appearance is normal. Oral mucosa is moist. Her lips are normal.
Her neck is supple, without adenopathy. Her heartbeat is regular with no
murmurs. Her lungs are clear. Her abdomen is soft and nontender. You
note no joint swelling or tenderness. Her skin demonstrates a diffuse
erythema with a finely bumpy rash (1 mm papules with prominent follicles). It is most bumpy over her back. It is slightly red over her face on
the cheeks, but this rash is smooth. There is a slightly reddish hue to the
rash, but because her skin pigmentation is dark, this is difficult to fully
appreciate. No urticarial lesions are seen.

Figure 23-1 illustrates her back, including her left shoulder, revealing the
reddish hue well. The rash is also slightly bumpy. Figure 23-2, which is
overexposed, is a photograph of her back; the bumpiness is best seen in
the lower right portion. A slight reddish hue (which looks pink in Figure
23-2) can be appreciated.

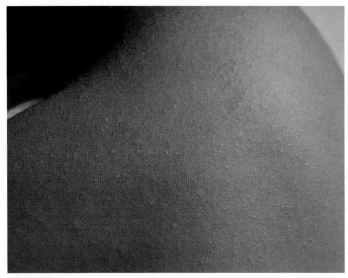

Figure 23-1

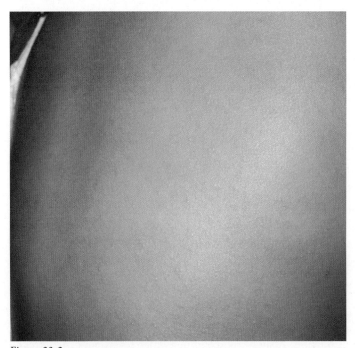

Figure 23-2

Discussion

Differential Diagnosis
- Scarlet fever
- Streptococcal pharyngitis with fever
- Viral pharyngitis

Evaluation
You obtain a rapid streptococcal throat swab assay, and it returns positive for group A streptococci. You diagnose her with scarlet fever.

Treatment
She is treated with penicillin and antipyretics.

Keep in Mind

Scarlet fever is due to an exotoxin produced by group A beta-hemolytic streptococci (GABHS), also known as *Streptococcus pyogenes.* This particular exotoxin results in rash and erythroderma, but it appears to be relatively harmless clinically. An uncommon form of staphylococcal scarlet fever also exists.

The scarlet fever rash usually appears within 1 to 2 days of the symptoms of sore throat and fever. It tends to involve the neck, upper extremities, and torso. The red hue is magenta, similar to a mild sunburn. It is sometimes said to resemble sandpaper, but a more accurate description is that of fine goose bumps or chicken skin, with prominent follicles producing a slightly bumpy appearance that is more visible than palpable. The redness is often more intense in body creases (Pastia lines). The face is less involved, and on the face, the redness tends to be smooth rather than bumpy. A strawberry tongue is present in some patients. The rash fades with convalescence, and visible desquamation often results, especially around the nails.

Symptoms and signs of group A streptococcal infection, such as sore throat, fever, tonsillitis (sometimes exudative), palatal petechiae, and lymphadenopathy, will also often be present. However, as with all streptococcal pharyngitis episodes, many of these findings may be absent.

Group A beta-hemolytic streptococci remain sensitive to penicillin; however, varying degrees of erythromycin and clindamycin resistance are present.

An erythroderma associated with fever should bring to mind the consideration of toxic shock syndrome and Kawasaki disease. Toxic shock syndrome is most often associated with an infection with *Staphylococcus aureus,* although a streptococcal toxic shock syndrome also exists. The erythroderma is usually not bumpy. Toxic shock patients will often be weak and have subtle signs of early shock. In the era before varicella vaccine, acute varicella patients with impetigo secondarily infecting the open varicella lesions would often present with a febrile erythroderma. Distinguishing scarlet fever from toxic shock syndrome was quite a challenge. Assuming that these were scarlet fever cases ran the risk of missing an early toxic shock syndrome. The subtle cutaneous differences could not be easily relied on because the numerous varicella lesions would dominate the skin findings. Culturing these lesions often results in growing both GABHS and *S aureus.* One approach was to start parenteral antistaphylococcal and anti-GABHS treatment in the ED and monitor the patient for several hours. A patient who remained stable after prolonged observation most likely had erythroderma caused by scarlet fever, while any signs of cardiovascular instability prompted hospitalization and treatment for early toxic shock.

Kawasaki disease has more prominent eye, tongue, and lip findings. The rash of Kawasaki disease is more often similar to erythema multiforme, although the rash pattern is variable and is often called polymorphous.

Scarlet fever might seem to be less virulent than it has been in the past. However, it is also possible that some cases of toxic shock syndrome were mistakenly diagnosed as scarlet fever in the past. Toxic shock syndrome was characterized in 1978. Before that, patients with toxic shock syndrome were probably mistakenly thought to have a virulent form of scarlet fever.

Recommended Reading

Gerber MA. Group A *Streptococcus*. In: Kliegman RM, Behrman RE, Jenson HB, Stanton BF, eds. *Nelson Textbook of Pediatrics*. 18th ed. Int ed. Philadelphia, PA: WB Saunders; 2007:1135–1145

Hayden GF, Turner RB. Acute pharyngitis. In: Kliegman RM, Behrman RE, Jenson HB, Stanton BF, eds. *Nelson Textbook of Pediatrics*. 18th ed. Int ed. Philadelphia, PA: WB Saunders; 2007:1752–1753

Part 3
Allergies and Skin Reactions

Chin Laceration, Drug Allergy, and Medical Errors

Presentation

A 10-year-old boy seeks care for a chin laceration. He fell forward, struck his chin on the ground, and experienced a bleeding wound. His mother washed the wound at home, the bleeding subsided, and she brought him to the emergency department (ED). He is allergic to lidocaine, ibuprofen, and penicillin.

While taking the patient's history, the ED physician learns that during a repair of a scalp laceration using lidocaine local anesthesia at age 5, he developed hives and eye swelling and was treated with diphenhydramine and prednisone. In retrospect, he also developed an allergic reaction of lip swelling when a teething medication that contained benzocaine was applied to his gums as an infant. He was treated with diphenhydramine, although at the time, the reaction was thought to be due to a new fruit that he had eaten. He also developed eye swelling during an ophthalmology evaluation when proparacaine drops were placed in his eyes. He has not required any significant dental work, so his dentist has never had reason to administer lidocaine.

Examination reveals that vital signs are normal. Examination is significant for a 1.5-cm chin laceration. His mandible and dental examinations are normal.

Discussion

Differential Diagnosis
- Chin laceration
- Lidocaine allergy

Evaluation

The patient and his mother are placed in a treatment room. He is assigned to a nurse who notices that he has a chin laceration. The ED has a standing order for lidocaine, adrenaline, and tetracaine (LAT) gel to be placed on chin lacerations in triage. The ED nurse assumes that the triage nurse was busy and didn't do this. A vial of LAT gel is removed from the ED dispensing unit, and the nurse is preparing to apply it to the patient's chin when the mother reminds the nurse that the patient is allergic to lidocaine.

Treatment

True lidocaine allergy is very rare. Although many patients will identify a history of mouth swelling after administration of dental lidocaine, most of these are not true allergic reactions. Local anesthetics are generally classified as amide (eg, lidocaine, bupivacaine) or ester (eg, procaine, tetracaine, benzocaine, cocaine) local anesthetics. There is cross-sensitivity within these groups, but allergy to both groups is still possible.

This patient has some history to suggest that he is allergic to both groups of drugs. To repair his chin laceration, there are several options. One possibility is to premedicate him with diphenhydramine (and possibly prednisone) before administering lidocaine local anesthesia. This option could succeed but is not guaranteed to prevent an allergic reaction. Another option is to sedate him systemically with propofol or ketamine so that he will not require any local anesthesia, but this option is medically aggressive and carries the modest risk of deep sedation. Another option is to not suture his chin laceration, but rather to use a tissue adhesive or perform a closure with wound closure tapes.

Another option is to use diphenhydramine as a local anesthetic. Parenteral diphenhydramine 50 mg/mL is diluted 1:4 (1 mL of diphenhydramine added to 4 mL of saline) and infiltrated as a local anesthetic. Although infiltration might be more painful, it produces sufficient local anesthesia for suturing. Additionally, 50 mg of diphenhydramine is a large dose for most children, so the volume must be limited to a much lower total dose of diphenhydramine, or diluting it further might be required. Large lacerations might require more than this dose, in which case the option of deep sedation should be considered rather than risk a diphenhydramine overdose. A more recent reference recommends against this use of diphenhydramine because of infiltration pain and a risk of tissue necrosis.

Diphenhydramine is an unusual drug in that it has many different properties and indications.

- It is a local anesthetic. It can be used as described herein, and it is also used as an oral swish for painful mouth ulcers as a topical anesthetic.
- It is a sedative.
- It is an anticholinergic, often employed to reverse acute dystonic reactions.
- It has antinausea properties and in the past was commonly used as an antiemetic.
- It is an antitussive agent, found in some over-the-counter cough medications.
- It is an antihistamine.
- It is an antipruritic.

This patient also has a history of penicillin allergy. Patients with drug allergies often have allergies to more than one class of drug. Patients with a history of penicillin allergy are often not truly penicillin allergic. Penicillin products delivered intramuscularly can contain procaine or benzathine. Procaine is a local anesthetic and could be the cause of the allergy, rather than the penicillin.

In this case, diluted parenteral diphenhydramine was used to infiltrate the wound for local anesthesia. The wound was closed with absorbable sutures.

Keep in Mind

Medication errors associated with drug allergies are common. In many instances, systems have been established to decrease the likelihood of these errors. In this case, several opportunities to prevent the error were present, yet the error nearly occurred until the last line of defense—the patient's vigilant mother—stopped it. In many cases, the mother would not have known what was in the LAT gel, and she would not have stopped the error from occurring. In an effort to streamline laceration care, a standing order to administer LAT gel established a system that focused on the laceration at the expense of recognizing the lidocaine allergy. If LAT gel is a standing order, nurses must know that this preparation contains lidocaine as well as adrenaline and tetracaine, and that adrenaline is also called epinephrine. Allergy to any of the drugs in a combination preparation would contraindicate its administration. Many combination medications are available, and nurses must know each of the medications to check for allergies.

Work flow optimization often focuses on accelerating task completion rather than avoiding errors. In this case, the triage nurse noted that the patient was allergic to lidocaine and entered this in the medical record. But if the allergy is not noted prominently and the nurse's work flow did not facilitate recognizing drug allergies, this could be missed. In a paper charting system, the identification of a drug allergy should ideally prompt several actions—prominently displaying the drug allergy by applying an allergy band or allergy sticker to the patient, applying a large allergy sticker to the clip on the chart clipboard, and writing the allergy on the discharge form (so that this allergy is not forgotten at discharge time).

In the paper chart pictured in Figure 24-1, the penicillin allergy is documented in 2 places, the chart's allergy box and on the clip of the clipboard. The allergy is more likely to be noticed with the added large sticker on the clip of the clipboard than in the chart allergy box alone.

A computer medical record and order entry system should ideally be smart enough to contain programming that blocks the ordering of allergic medications. In this case, once the triage nurse entered the lidocaine allergy into the computer system, the automated drug dispensing unit should refuse to

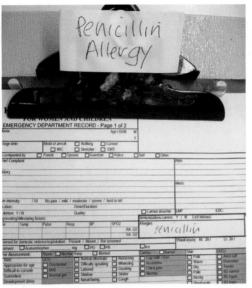

Figure 24-1

dispense LAT gel to the nurse because it should know about the patient's allergy. A smart computer system does not necessarily prevent all such errors. The intelligence level of the computer cannot always be ensured. Does the computer know that LAT contains lidocaine and it should block dispensing LAT for lidocaine-allergic patients? Is the computer smart enough to block dispensing Unasyn (ampicillin and sulbactam) for patients who are allergic to amoxicillin? Such complex algorithms must be programmed into the system. In other words, a human programmer must be able to anticipate the problem so that the computer can be programmed to block it.

In addition, the computer can be fooled in several ways. Even if the computer system knows that LAT contains lidocaine, perhaps a new physician looks for LET (lidocaine, epinephrine, tetracaine) in the computer's formulary drop-down list but can't find it, so the physician calls the pharmacist and asks if the hospital has LET gel. The pharmacist responds, "Yes." The physician enters the order as free text—"apply LET gel to wound." The computer knows that LAT contains lidocaine, but it has never heard of LET before.

As another example, a resident is told to order Unasyn 1 gram intravenous (IV) for the patient. The patient is allergic to ampicillin and amoxicillin. This resident has never ordered Unasyn for a patient before, so he doesn't know that it contains ampicillin. He thinks the drug is spelled "unison" and he can't find it in the computer's formulary drop-down list, so he simply enters it in free text as "unison 1 gram IV." The pharmacist realizes that this is Unasyn. Hopefully, the pharmacist has recognized the ampicillin drug allergy, because the computer system has missed it due to the misspelling of the drug's name.

Recommended Reading

deShazo RD, Nelson HS. An approach to the patient with a history of local anesthetic hypersensitivity: experience with 90 patients. *J Allergy Clin Immunol.* 1979;63:387–394

Ernst AA, Anand P, Nick T, Wassmuth S. Lidocaine versus diphenhydramine for anesthesia in the repair of minor lacerations. *J Trauma.* 1993;34:354–357

Ernst AA, Marvez-Valls E, Mall G, Patterson J, Xie X, Weiss SJ. 1% lidocaine versus 0.5% diphenhydramine for local anesthesia in minor laceration repair. *Ann Emerg Med.* 1994;23:1328–1332

Ernst AA, Marvez-Valls E, Nick TG, Wahle M. Comparison trial of four injectable anesthetics for laceration repair. *Acad Emerg Med.* 1996;3:228–233

Incaudo G, Schatz M, Patterson R, Rosenberg M, Yamamoto F, Hamburger RN. Administration of local anesthetics to patients with a history of prior adverse reaction. *J Allergy Clin Immunol.* 1978;61:339–345

Pollack CV, Swindle GM. Use of diphenhydramine for local anesthesia in "caine"-sensitive patients. *J Emerg Med.* 1989;7:611–614

Selby SM, Fein JA. Sedation and analgesia. In: Fleisher GR, Ludwig S, Henretig FM, Ruddy RM, Silverman BK, eds. *Textbook of Pediatric Emergency Medicine.* 5th ed. Philadelphia, PA: Lippincott Williams & Wilkins; 2006:70

Chapter 25

Rash With Peeling

Presentation

An almost 2-year-old girl arrives at the emergency department (ED) on the second day of an illness characterized by a painful erythroderma. Her mother reports that the rash began around the mouth and progressed to the trunk and perineum. She underwent an evaluation at a different ED the previous night. She has since developed periorificial cracking and peeling on the chest where monitor leads had been placed. The patient has been fussy and her skin appears tender to touch everywhere. She has had no fevers or vomiting and, despite her discomfort, is eating well. She was previously healthy and takes no medications.

Her vital signs include the following: temperature 37.5°C, heart rate 148 beats/min, and respiratory rate 36 breaths/min. She is fussy but easily consoled. She is alert and makes appropriate eye contact. Perioral erythema and fissuring is present (Figure 25-1), but there is no oral mucosal or conjunctival involvement. Genital examination reveals erythema and desquamation of the labia majora bilaterally. Skin examination is notable for a diffuse truncal erythroderma with several regions of desquamation on the anterior chest (Figure 25-2). There is no palmar or plantar involvement, and no apparent primary focus of infection.

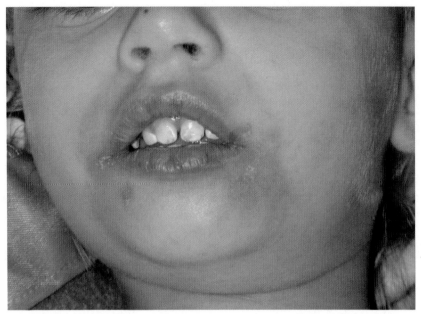

Figure 25-1

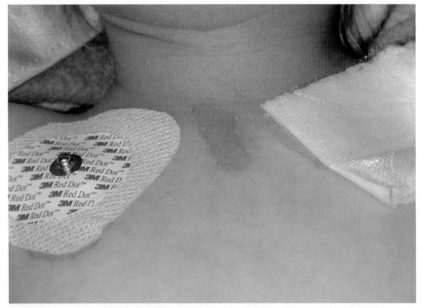

Figure 25-2

Discussion

Differential Diagnosis
- Scarlet fever
- Stevens-Johnson syndrome
- Toxic epidermal necrolysis
- Thermal or chemical injury
- Staphylococcal scalded skin syndrome (SSSS)
- Kawasaki disease

Evaluation
The evaluation is based primarily on clinical diagnosis. Screening tests make inflammatory conditions such as Stevens-Johnson syndrome or Kawasaki disease unlikely. The white blood cell count is 13,600/μL, hemoglobin 12.6 g/dL, platelets 435,000/μL, and C-reactive protein less than 0.7 mg/dL. Electrolytes are normal.

Treatment
This manifestation is most consistent with SSSS with no evidence of other serious problems. Because the patient sought care early in the disease course and appears well hydrated, a plan is established with the primary physician for parenteral antibiotics in the ED followed by oral antibiotics and close outpatient follow-up. The patient receives a dose of intravenous (IV) cefazolin in the ED with outpatient prescriptions for cephalexin and acetaminophen-codeine. She does well initially, but 3 days later, she develops increased pain and erythema as well as fever (temperature to 39.0°C). She returns to your ED with progression of bullous lesions. She receives IV hydration, clindamycin, and analgesics. After admission, her antibiotic therapy is continued with clindamycin, and after 2 hospital days, pain and fever begin to improve. The patient receives IV fluid rehydration until her oral intake improves. Cultures of nares, blood, and urine remain negative at the time of discharge.

Keep in Mind

Staphylococcal scalded skin syndrome is a clinical diagnosis. Tender erythroderma and perioral radial fissuring are characteristic. The most important distinction to make in the ED setting is with toxic epidermal necrolysis, which has a greater morbidity and mortality and which may benefit from therapy with IV immunoglobulin.

The skin lesions result from dissemination of exfoliative toxin produced at a distant site of staphylococcal infection. The blisters themselves are sterile. The exfoliative toxin cleaves desmoglein 1, an intercellular adhesion molecule, only in the superficial epidermis. Although seldom necessary, this localization permits histologic differentiation from toxic epidermal necrolysis, which involves a deeper dermal-epidermal separation.

Supportive care is directed at correcting fluid balance and achieving pain relief. Empiric therapy with antistaphylococcal therapy is appropriate, and traditionally first-generation cephalosporins or penicillinase-resistant penicillins such as dicloxacillin were recommended. In this case, outpatient therapy with an oral cephalosporin was unsuccessful. Although the pathogen infecting this patient was not identified, emergence of methicillin resistance in conjunction with staphylococcal scalded skin syndrome makes consideration of antibiotic therapy directed against methicillin-resistant *Staphylococcus aureus* (MRSA) prudent. Although MRSA remains much less common in SSSS than in skin and soft tissue infections, many experts no longer recommend empiric therapy with a beta-lactam antibiotic. Agents that inhibit bacterial protein synthesis, such as clindamycin and linezolid, offer the potential advantage of reducing toxin production. In all cases of suspected staphylococcal infection, initial antibiotic therapy should be directed by current knowledge of the local prevalence of MRSA and of the frequency of clindamycin resistance and clindamycin-inducible resistance among MRSA isolates. Vancomycin may be required in life-threatening infections or when the community prevalence of clindamycin resistance is high.

Recommended Reading

American Academy of Pediatrics. Staphylococcal infections. In: Pickering LK, Baker CJ, Kimberlin DW, Long SS, eds. *Red Book: 2009 Report of the Committee on Infectious Diseases.* 28th ed. Elk Grove Village, IL: American Academy of Pediatrics; 2009:601–615

Paller AS, Mancini AJ. Bacterial, mycobacterial, and protozoal infections of the skin. In: *Hurwitz Clinical Pediatric Dermatology: A Textbook of Skin Disorders of Childhood and Adolescence.* 3rd ed. Philadelphia, PA: Elsevier Saunders; 2006;365–395

Stanley JR, Amagai M. Pemphigus, bullous impetigo, and the staphylococcal scalded-skin syndrome. *N Engl J Med.* 2006;355:1800–1810

Chapter 26

Hives Resistant to Diphenhydramine

Presentation

A 4-year-old boy with a history of vesicoureteral reflux sought care at the emergency department (ED) yesterday with dysuria of 6 hours' duration. There is no history of fever or vomiting. A clean-catch urinalysis showed 50 to 100 white blood cells per high-power field. A diagnosis of urinary tract infection was made, and he was discharged with trimethoprim-sulfamethoxazole (Bactrim, Septra). His parents noticed an alarming rash this morning. They gave him a dose of diphenhydramine, but the rash did not improve, so they brought him back to the ED. Yesterday's urine culture has grown 100,000 gram-negative rod colonies per mL.

Past medical history includes vesicoureteral reflux that is improving, and his parents stopped his antibiotic prophylaxis 1 month ago without telling his doctor. Social history is negative. Family history reveals that the patient's 5-year-old brother has a cold. The child's immunizations are up to date.

Examination reveals the following vital signs: tympanic temperature 37.2°C, pulse 80 beats/min, respiration 25 breaths/min, and blood pressure 90/55 mm Hg. He is alert, active, and smiling, and he is in no distress. Eyes reveal mild conjunctival injection. Tympanic membranes are normal. There are no lesions in his oral mucosa, which is moist. His lips are normal. His neck is supple without adenopathy. His heartbeat is regular with no murmurs, and his lungs are clear. He is not coughing. There is no tachypnea. His abdomen is soft and nontender with normal, active bowel sounds. There are no inguinal hernias. External genitalia are normal; he has been circumcised. He moves all extremities well. His facial motor function is good.

The rash is very prominent. There are large and small areas of raised ery-thematous patches of various shapes. His mother indicates that she thinks that the rash itches and some of the lesions have moved from one part of the body to another. Some lesions exhibit central clearing—that is, they resemble targets. Examination of the medial left upper arm reveals the different shapes and irregular borders of the rash (Figure 26-1). His right forearm has lesions of varying sizes and shapes; some lesions are slightly elevated with slight depression of the central portion of the lesion (Figure 26-2). His right lateral chest contains target lesions (circles) and has patches of various shapes and sizes (Figure 26 3).

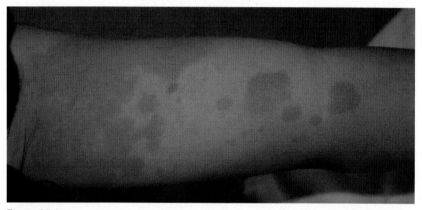

Figure 26-1

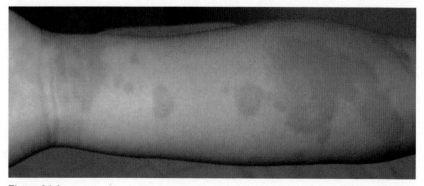

Figure 26-2

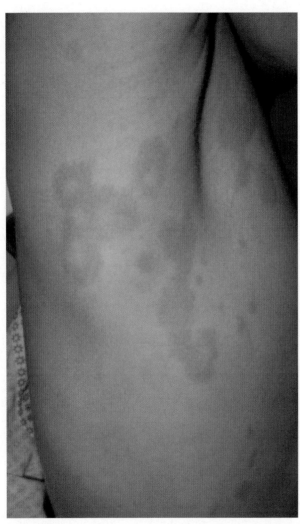

Figure 26-3

Discussion

Differential Diagnosis
- Erythema multiforme minor
- Erythema multiforme major (Stevens-Johnson syndrome [SJS])
- Kawasaki disease
- Urinary tract infection

Evaluation
Erythema multiforme is often a type 3 hypersensitivity reaction (immune complex mediated). Although the rash of erythema multiforme frequently resembles urticaria, several clinical clues help to distinguish the two. Erythema multiforme is resistant to treatment with antihistamines. A frequent chief complaint is that a patient with hives is treated with diphenhydramine but the hives do not resolve. Most urticaria (type 1 hypersensitivity) is histamine mediated, and resolution occurs promptly after treatment with an antihistamine. However, most studies on the treatment of erythema multiforme indicate that the response to antihistamines (H1 or H2 receptor antagonists) is minimal at best. Most cases of erythema multiforme will resolve over 1 to 2 weeks or longer.

As in this patient, parents will often describe erythema multiforme lesions as migrating to different parts of the body and their shapes as changing. In addition, many patients with erythema multiforme develop arthritis of the hands and feet manifested by joint swelling and an unwillingness to walk. This will resolve, but parents should be advised of this so that when it occurs, an unnecessary visit to the ED can be avoided.

Erythema multiforme minor is the more common presentation. Erythema multiforme major implies the involvement of mucosal surfaces (ie, mouth, lips, gastrointestinal tract, genitourinary tract, and conjunctiva). In this case, the patient has mild conjunctival injection, but his oral mucosa and lips are normal. Erythema multiforme major is also called SJS. The most severe form along the continuum of SJS is toxic epidermal necrolysis, which results in severe sloughing of the skin and mucosal surfaces. Toxic epidermal necrolysis has a high mortality rate. This patient could potentially have an early and mild case of SJS because of the mild conjunctival injection; however, involvement of the other mucosal surfaces is not present.

Kawasaki disease is known to have fever, a polymorphous rash (which includes erythema multiforme), and conjunctival injection. However, this patient lacks the associated oral mucosal and lip abnormalities. Febrile patients with erythema multiforme should be evaluated or followed clinically for the possibility of Kawasaki disease.

In this case, the cause of the erythema multiforme is most likely sulfon-amide antibiotics; however, in most instances, the cause cannot be iden-tified. Occult food allergies might be the cause. A dietary recall history in most instances does not yield any new foods. Other known associations of erythema multiforme include herpes simplex, mycoplasma, and group A streptococcus.

Treatment
Treatment of erythema multiforme minor is limited. Antihistamines (H1 and H2 receptor antagonists) and corticosteroids have not been shown to help. Pruritus can be reduced, but not eliminated, with some antihista-mines or topical agents. This patient's parents were advised that treatment for this condition is limited, but to expect this to gradually resolve on its own in about 2 weeks.

Keep in Mind
Sulfonamide antibiotics such as trimethoprim-sulfamethoxazole are inexpensive and highly efficacious. However, sulfonamides have 2 major concerns. Sulfonamides may result in a higher risk of SJS—an important potential adverse event about which doctors should advise patients. The other concern is that if the patient has glucose-6-phosphate dehydrogenase (G6PD) deficiency, sulfonamides can cause an acute hemolytic reaction. Because G6PD deficiency is occult in many patients and because patients with known G6PD deficiency may not mention this condition, before prescribing sulfonamides the physician should inquire specifically about a family history of G6PD deficiency.

Recommended Reading

Gruskin KD. Rash—maculopapular. In: Fleisher GR, Ludwig S, Henretig
    FM, Ruddy RM, Silverman BK, eds. *Textbook of Pediatric Emergency
    Medicine.* 5th ed. Philadelphia, PA: Lippincott Williams & Wilkins;
    2006:559–570

Morelli JG. Vesiculobullous disorders. In: Kliegman RM, Behrman RE,
    Jenson HB, Stanton BF, eds. *Nelson Textbook of Pediatrics.* 18th ed.
    Int ed. Philadelphia, PA: WB Saunders; 2007:2685–2693

Chapter 27

Peanut Allergy

Presentation

A 10-year-old girl is brought to the emergency department (ED) by ambulance because of wheezing. She was dropped off at soccer practice in the afternoon. Today, one of the parents served the children a chili snack and drinks during practice. The girl was eating some chili when she developed facial swelling, difficulty breathing, and weakness. A parent called 911. When the ambulance arrived, the paramedics administered subcutaneous epinephrine, and an albuterol nebulizer treatment was initiated. An intravenous line was started, and she was transported to the ED.

The patient's past medical history is significant for mild asthma and for peanut and tree nut allergies. She has required treatment with epinephrine, antihistamines, and corticosteroids on 3 previous occasions. Her previous episodes were similar—they were all characterized by facial swelling, urticaria, and wheezing. She has never had an episode of loss of consciousness or known hypotension. Her mother carries an epinephrine injector, and she has given one to the school nurse.

Examination reveals the following vital signs: oral temperature 36.6°C, pulse 95 beats/min, respiration 25 breaths/min, blood pressure 105/75 mm Hg, and oxygen saturation 100% on supplemental oxygen. She is alert, active, and cooperative and appears to be in no acute distress. She has mild periorbital edema. Her conjunctivae are clear and not edematous. Her tympanic membranes are normal. Her lips are not swollen. Her pharynx is normal. Her heartbeat is regular without murmurs, and her lungs are clear with good aeration. Her abdomen is soft and nontender. Her skin shows some fading urticaria. Her overall perfusion is good.

Discussion

Differential Diagnosis
- Peanut allergy hypersensitivity reaction consisting of bronchospasm and urticaria

Evaluation
She is stable for now, but her allergic reaction history is severe. Patients with peanut allergy often require aggressive treatment with epinephrine and other antiallergy medications.

Treatment
Intravenous diphenhydramine and methylprednisolone are administered. She is observed in the ED for 5 hours with orthostatic blood pressure checks. Her status remains stable. She is now ambulatory without any light-headedness or weakness. She is discharged with antihistamines and oral corticosteroids. Her family lives close by and her parents are capable observers.

Keep in Mind

The term *anaphylaxis* is defined as an exaggerated allergic reaction. This results in some vagueness because severe urticaria could be included in this. Should bronchospasm and mild wheezing be considered anaphylaxis? Most would agree that cardiovascular collapse with hypotension qualifies as anaphylaxis. But where anaphylaxis starts is vague. Thus, if the term anaphylaxis is to be used, it should be further qualified, such as "anaphylaxis with wheezing and mild light-headedness without confirmed hypotension." This is much clearer than anaphylaxis by itself.

Nut allergies are generally categorized into peanuts and tree nuts. Peanuts grow underground, whereas most other nuts grow on trees. Some patients are allergic to peanuts and tree nuts. Peanut allergy is generally thought to be the most serious food allergy. Treatment with epinephrine is often necessary and highly recommended in all cases because better outcomes have been demonstrated with early epinephrine treatment.

Peanut allergy and most food allergies present substantial life-changing compromises and risks. It is extremely difficult to avoid exposure to these allergens because they are ubiquitous and often hidden. Children require vigilant parental supervision. This is a serious and significant challenge for teens exploring their newfound independence.

Food allergens are often hidden. For example, which of the following contain peanuts or tree nuts? Cosmetic facial scrub; muffins; Chinese egg rolls; chili; hot chocolate; apple pie; breakfast cereal; salsa; furniture beanbags; pet foods; Asian restaurants (especially Chinese, Thai, Vietnamese, and Indonesian cooking); Mexican restaurants; ice cream; steel ball bearings.

Except for ball bearings, all of the above could contain peanuts or other nuts. Cosmetic abrasive facial scrubs often contain ground walnut shells. Muffins often contain ground nuts or nut products. Chinese egg rolls contain peanut oil and peanut sauces. Chili contains peanut products. Hot chocolate contains nut products. Many pastries and cereals are made with nut products. Salsa and some Mexican foods contain nut products. Furniture beanbags may contain nut shells. Pet foods contain nut products to increase their protein content. Asian restaurants often cook with peanut oil and other nut oils. Ice cream can be easily contaminated at buffets and ice cream parlors by nut residue used on sundaes and other preparations.

School and other social activities (like this patient's soccer snacks) place food allergy patients at risk because the parents who have prepared the foods are not aware of the food allergy. Most parents do not understand the pervasive nature of food ingredients that place allergic patients at risk for reactions. Cookies, chili, ice cream, cakes, pastries, and sandwiches may all place food-allergic patients at significant risk. Children are generally not capable of avoiding all allergic foods, and parents cannot be present with their children 100% of the time.

Food labels are deceiving. For example, "nondairy" coffee whitener still contains milk proteins. Egg substitutes still contain egg proteins.

The topic of food allergies is underappreciated by many physicians. A thorough discussion of management and food avoidance for a particular food allergy is beyond the scope of time available for a typical ED visit.

Referring patients to an allergist or a reliable informational Internet resource such as www.foodallergy.org is often a useful way to provide patients and their families with more information.

Epinephrine injection kits should be provided to parents of children with peanut allergy. However, it should be appreciated that administering an injection to one's child is an intimidating task for a parent who has never done this before, even though practice devices are available. Autoinjectors like the EpiPen simplify this process. Additionally, the epinephrine injector must be carried by a parent at all times for it to be available when the need arises. It must also be available when the parent is not present, such as while the child is in school.

Recommended Reading

Sampson HA, Muñoz-Furlong A, Campbell RL, et al. Second symposium on the definition and management of anaphylaxis: summary report—second National Institute of Allergy and Infectious Disease/Food Allergy and Anaphylaxis Network symposium. *Ann Emerg Med.* 2006;47:373–380

Thatayatikom A. Food allergies. In: Yamamoto LG, Inaba AS, Okamoto JK, Patronis ME, Yamashiroya VK, eds. *Case Based Pediatrics for Medical Students and Residents.* Honolulu, HI: University of Hawaii; 2004:126–130. Available at: http://www.hawaii.edu/medicine/pediatrics/pedtext. Accessed December 17, 2008

Chapter 28

Outbreak of Hives

Presentation

A school nurse calls the emergency department (ED) with the news that she is sending 10 schoolchildren to the ED because of an outbreak of hives. She tells you that a child was sent to her with hives and she gave the child diphenhydramine. Five minutes later, she received 2 other children from a different classroom with hives, and before she could administer treatment, she received 4 other children with hives. She told the school principal that something odd was occurring because it is not typical for so many children to have hives at once. She advised the principal to have all of the children taken to the ED for evaluation. A total of 10 children with hives are now being sent to the ED. Three cars bring the 10 children to the ED.

Past medical histories are variable but largely negative.

At physical examination, vital signs are normal. All children have similar findings during their examinations. They are alert, active, and itchy. Their faces are red and they have urticarial lesions over many parts of their bodies. Heart and lung examinations are normal. No respiratory distress is noted.

Discussion

Differential Diagnosis
- Scombroid poisoning
- A coincidental cluster of urticaria

Evaluation
Further history reveals that a teacher also developed hives. He has a history of hives, so he took a loratadine tablet as soon as he felt itchy, and his symptoms resolved.

The school lunch is prepared by school cafeteria staff. Baked fish (mahi-mahi, also known as dolphin fish) was served today. Scombroid poisoning is suspected.

Treatment
All 10 children are deemed to be stable. The one child who was given diphenhydramine is clearly improved compared with the other children. The other 9 children are given oral diphenhydramine and are observed in the ED. After 2 hours, the redness and urticaria are much better. Vital signs remain normal, and they are discharged from the ED into the care of their parents.

Keep in Mind
Histidine is one of the amino acids contained in proteins. Some marine fish contain disproportionally large amounts of histidine. If the flesh of the fish decays during the process of harvesting, transport, or storage, the histidine is metabolized to histamine, so it's important that the fish be immediately iced. The term *scombroid poisoning* originates from this group of fish, known as scombroid fish (eg, tuna, mackerel, swordfish) (Figure 28-1). However, other fish such as mahimahi have also been known to cause scombroid poisoning.

Scombroid poisoning essentially results from ingesting large amounts of histamine. This histamine can trigger urticaria or the more serious manifestations of type 1 hypersensitivity reactions such as bronchospasm, laryngeal edema, orthostatic hypotension, and cardiovascular collapse.

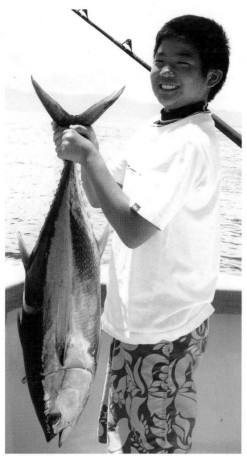

Patients have been successfully treated with H1 and H2 blockers, both of which can be given orally or intravenously. Intravenous administration is preferred for patients who have intravenous access and who are more seriously ill. Epinephrine can be used to treat the more serious cardiovascular or airway symptoms.

Figure 28-1

Recommended Reading

Osterhoudt KC, Ewald MB, Shannon M, Henretig FM. Toxicologic emergencies. In: Fleisher GR, Ludwig S, Henretig FM, Ruddy RM, Silverman BK, eds. *Textbook of Pediatric Emergency Medicine.* 5th ed. Philadelphia, PA: Lippincott Williams & Wilkins; 2006:951–1007

Salerno DA, Aronoff SC. Nonbacterial food poisoning. In: Kliegman RM, Behrman RE, Jenson HB, Stanton BF, eds. *Nelson Textbook of Pediatrics.* 18th ed. Int ed. Philadelphia, PA: WB Saunders; 2007:2918–2919

Chapter 29

Egg Allergy, Radioallergosorbent Test, and Propofol

Presentation

A 10-month-old boy is brought to the emergency department (ED) by ambulance after being attacked by his uncle's dog. He was playing with the dog when the dog unexpectedly attacked the child, biting him on his face several times. A lot of bleeding was noted, and 911 was called. The paramedics started an intravenous (IV) line en route. No loss of consciousness occurred; the child was crying when the paramedics arrived. A radio order for morphine was given, and now he is more calm and comfortable.

Past medical history is negative. The child does not have asthma or drug allergies, and his immunizations are up to date.

Examination reveals the following vital signs: axillary temperature 36.5°C, pulse 105 beats/min, respiration 25 breaths/min, and blood pressure 105/80 mm Hg. He is awake, alert, cooperative, and comfortable. There are many large, deep lacerations over both cheeks and his lips, crossing through the vermillion border. There are no scalp, eye, or ear injuries. Heart, lungs, and abdomen are normal. There are no extremity or torso wounds. Overall color and perfusion are good.

Discussion

Differential Diagnosis
• Multiple facial dog bite wounds

Evaluation
Because this child's wounds are fairly extensive, sedation during wound repair would be optimal. The time since the patient last ate should be ascertained. If the patient just ate a full meal, it is safer to wait. Drug allergies, history (especially anesthesia or sedation history), and current or recent ill symptoms should be ascertained.

Treatment
Treatment for pain was addressed en route with the order for morphine; more can be given IV as needed. Antibiotics are given promptly; penicillin or ampicillin should be given to cover *Pasteurella multocida*. In the past, cephalosporins would be given to cover *Staphylococcus aureus,* but the prevalence of methicillin-resistant *S aureus* (MRSA) in the community is increasing, so clindamycin or another appropriate anti-MRSA drug is given instead. Clindamycin and penicillin also cover anaerobes well.

A plastic surgeon is called to repair the infant's wounds. The plastic surgeon requests that the patient be sedated so that the wounds can be best repaired, and the parents agree. An additional ED physician is called in to perform the sedation because hospital regulations require a credentialed physician to be continuously present during deep sedation. The on-duty ED physician has other patients to see and cannot meet this requirement.

The second ED physician arrives and interviews the family, and together they decide on the best sedation. The 3 most common choices in this instance are propofol, ketamine, or etomidate. Ketamine has analgesic properties that give it an advantage, but ketamine has a longer recovery time, there is a risk of laryngospasm and excessive oral secretions, and there is a higher frequency of vomiting. Propofol has no analgesic properties, but the patient can be deeply sedated or sedated in conjunction with a narcotic analgesic. Propofol has the advantage of a shorter recovery time and fewer adverse effects on awakening. After weighing the advantages and disadvantages, the ED physician and parents decide that the best choice is propofol. Etomidate is not considered in this case.

Propofol contains egg proteins and soybean oil, so patients who are allergic to eggs or soy should not receive propofol. Asthma is not an absolute contraindication to propofol, but a history of severe asthma might shift the balance of clinical factors to favor ketamine because ketamine has bronchodilator properties. This patient has no known drug allergies or history of asthma. However, when the physician specifically asks whether he has eaten eggs or soy products before, an interesting reply is provided by his parents.

His current infant formula is a soy formula, so it is unlikely that he is allergic to soy products. His parents did give him some scrambled eggs once, and they noticed that his upper lip became modestly swollen. This resolved on its own, and he did not have any hives or experience any respiratory symptoms. They told his pediatrician about this, and his pediatrician ordered a blood test to see whether he was allergic to eggs. Although the test results indicated that he is not allergic to eggs, they have not given him eggs since.

At this point, the physician decides that the patient might be allergic to eggs and decides to use ketamine instead. The patient is sedated with atropine and ketamine. The plastic surgeon repairs his wounds. He recovers uneventfully in the ED. He is discharged with oral amoxicillin and clindamycin.

Keep in Mind

Although many reports in the literature have been published concluding that sedation in the ED is safe, this doesn't mean that this safety record is achieved easily. Propofol and ketamine are deep sedatives, and the person performing the sedation must be able to rescue the patient from any airway compromise. Trained ED physicians must have the skills to manage an airway emergency. These skills include bag-mask ventilation, airway manipulation and repositioning, and tracheal intubation.

Additionally, the potential adverse effects of these drugs should be well known by physicians who use them. In this particular case, an allergy to eggs was suspected, and the physician decided to avoid propofol. This infant had a single episode of lip swelling when he ate a small amount of scrambled eggs. Propofol contains egg products, and it is administered IV. The potential for a more serious allergic reaction contraindicates its use.

The patient's history revealed that a "blood test" had been performed to test the patient for egg allergy. This mostly likely was a radioallergosorbent test (RAST) study. This blood test measures immunoglobulin E levels against specific allergens. In this case, a food-allergy egg RAST study was probably ordered. The problem with RAST studies is that the probability of food allergy is dependent on the test result, the specific allergen, and the brand of the RAST study ordered. Most RAST assays are not standardized, so that probability tables for one brand of RAST study do not apply to another brand of RAST study. Using the wrong probability values could result in a high false-positive rate and false-negative rate. For example, for one particular brand of RAST products, an egg RAST value below 0.35 indicates that there is a 95% probability that the patient is not allergic to eggs. This means that one out of 20 patients who test "negative" for egg allergy are actually truly allergic to eggs. If the egg RAST value is greater than 7, there is 95% chance that the patient is truly allergic to eggs. This means that the false-positive rate is one in 20. Intermediate RAST levels are fairly nondiagnostic. Suffice it to say that there are many difficulties with properly interpreting RAST results. Extreme values of RAST assays might be helpful, but a negative RAST does not always rule out food allergy.

Egg hypersensitivity and propofol contraindications are more complex. Most patients allergic to eggs are allergic to the egg white (ovalbumin); however, propofol contains egg lecithin components found in the egg yolk. This reduces the risk of propofol hypersensitivity in egg-allergic patients. Clinicians must weight the advantages of propofol over the potential adverse effects of propofol in egg-allergic children in determining whether to use propofol or an alternate agent.

In this case, the family was told that the child was not allergic to eggs. Although this seems to be only a minor misstatement, it could have resulted in a reaction to propofol. Lip swelling after eating eggs is a convincing sign that the child is allergic to something that touched his lips. If the only new food was eggs, it should take more than a negative RAST study to rule out an egg allergy.

Recommended Reading

Hepner DL, Castells MC. Anaphylaxis during the perioperative period. *Anesth Analg.* 2003;97:1381–1395

Sacchetti A. Procedural sedation and analgesia. In: Gausche-Hill M, Fuchs S, Yamamoto L, eds. *APLS: The Pediatric Emergency Medicine Resource.* 4th rev ed. Sudbury, MA: Jones and Bartlett Publishers; 2007:498–523

Thatayatikom A. Food allergies. In: Yamamoto LG, Inaba AS, Okamoto JK, Patronis ME, Yamashiroya VK, eds. *Case Based Pediatrics for Medical Students and Residents.* Honolulu, HI: University of Hawaii; 2004:126–130. Available at: http://www.hawaii.edu/medicine/pediatrics/pedtext. Accessed December 17, 2008

Chapter 30

Bloody Stool and Pallor

Presentation

A 6-year-old girl developed abdominal pain and bloody stools 1 week before her mother brings her to the emergency department (ED). She was assessed at another hospital the day after the onset of her symptoms, and there she was found to be afebrile and to have a blood pressure of 114/73 mm Hg and hemoglobin 13.0 g/dL. She received fluid hydration and prescriptions for belladonna-phenobarbital and trimethoprim-sulfamethoxazole for a presumed diagnosis of bacterial enteritis.

Because she failed to improve, her family sought care nearby in Mexico and received a metronidazole-iodoquinol combination and a *Lactobacillus*-containing supplement. Bloody stools continued to occur twice daily with the consistency of applesauce. Now, on this visit to the ED, family members note that she is becoming progressively more pale. They have not noticed changes in her urine output. They deny ill contacts, and she has been afebrile and has had no respiratory symptoms.

She has a low-grade fever (temperature 38.0°C) and is slightly tachycardic (121 beats/min) but normotensive (111/68 mm Hg). She is alert with normal mental status and age-appropriate behavior, but she is pale. She does not have jaundice. Her conjunctivae are pale but anicteric. Her abdomen is soft with no guarding, masses, or hepatosplenomegaly. She has no adenopathy. Her skin examination is notable for marked pallor, but you note no rash or unusual bruising.

Discussion

Differential Diagnosis

- Gastrointestinal hemorrhage (eg, Meckel diverticulum, ulcer, esophageal varices)
- Trauma
- Bacterial enteritis
- Primary coagulopathy
- Intussusception
- Neoplasm (leukemia)
- Hemolytic uremic syndrome (HUS)

Evaluation

Laboratory studies include white blood cells 14,600/µL (54% segmented neutrophils, 12% band forms, 28% lymphocytes, and 5% monocytes), hemoglobin 7.1 g/dL, platelet count 23,000/µL, potassium 3.8 mmol/L, blood urea nitrogen (BUN) 122 mg/dL, and creatinine 3.6 mg/dL. The peripheral blood smear contains schistocytes but no cells are suspicious for malignancy. Prothrombin time and partial thromboplastin time are normal at 12.4 and 24 seconds, respectively.

Treatment

Although urine output has not changed, the impressive azotemia, together with thrombocytopenia with evidence of hemolytic anemia, make HUS the most likely cause.

During her ED stay, the patient's vital signs remain stable with normal blood pressure. She is admitted to a monitored inpatient setting for supportive care and observation. Despite the anemia, the initial plan is to delay transfusion while monitoring her hemoglobin closely. During the 7-day hospital stay, her hemoglobin reaches a nadir of 5.4 g/dL, resulting in transfusions on 2 occasions. Her platelet count decreases to 19,000/µL before beginning to increase, and her BUN and creatinine progressively improve with intravenous hydration, with values at discharge of 18 mg/dL and 0.5 mg/dL, respectively. No oligoanuria or mental status changes occur. Stool cultures yield no pathogens.

Keep in Mind

Hemolytic uremic syndrome is the most common cause of renal failure in children, particularly in children younger than 3 years. Diagnosis is based on the triad of microangiopathic hemolytic anemia, thrombocytopenia, and renal insufficiency. Most cases are associated with diarrhea (D+ HUS) typically caused by verotoxin (or Shiga-like toxin) producing enterohemorrhagic *Escherichia coli* O157:H7. Non-O157 strains and invasive pneumococcal infections also cause HUS. Hemolytic uremic syndrome without diarrhea (D- HUS) is associated with various drugs, medical conditions, and infections.

The typical preceding infection is characterized by abdominal pain with bloody diarrhea, often without fever. Only a small number of patients with *E coli* O157:H7 go on to develop HUS, typically after resolution of the diarrheal illness. Nearly half of these will experience oligoanuria requiring dialysis. Central nervous system pathology occurs in 20% and may include confusion, seizures, cerebral edema, and encephalopathy. Mortality in D+ HUS is 3%, and 30% of survivors experience some degree of long-term renal disease.

Bloody diarrhea should prompt screening for *E coli* O157:H7, and close attention must be paid to hydration status, urine output, and the development of pallor if the organism is isolated. Intravenously administered isotonic fluid during the diarrheal illness may reduce the risk of oligoanuric renal failure if HUS subsequently develops. Antimotility agents increase the risk of progression to HUS and its neurologic sequelae. Controversy exists regarding the role of antibiotic therapy in *E coli* O157 infection and the risk of subsequent HUS. The most effective measure against Shiga-toxin–producing *E coli* infection and HUS is prevention by careful food handling and preparation practices.

Recommended Reading

Cohen AR. Pallor. In: Fleisher GR, Ludwig S, Henretig FM, Ruddy RM, Silverman BK, eds. *Textbook of Pediatric Emergency Medicine.* 5th ed. Philadelphia, PA: Lippincott Williams & Wilkins; 2006:535–543

Loirat C, Taylor CM. Hemolytic uremic syndromes. In: Avner ED, Harmon WE, Niaudet P, eds. *Pediatric Nephrology.* 5th ed. Philadelphia, PA: Lippincott Williams & Wilkins; 2004:885–915

Serna A, Boedeker EC. Pathogenesis and treatment of Shiga toxin–producing Escherichia coli infections. *Curr Opin Gastroenterol.* 2008;24:38–47

Siegler R, Oakes R. Hemolytic uremic syndrome; pathogenesis, treatment, and outcome. *Curr Opin Pediatr.* 2005;17:200–204

Part 4

Injuries

Chapter 31

Severe Pain While Swimming

Presentation

A 14-year-old girl presents to the emergency department (ED) with severe pain to her left shoulder, back, and chest. She was swimming in the ocean at 7:00 am and suddenly felt severe pain in the area. She did not feel anything hit her or bite her. A lifeguard sprinkled vinegar and meat tenderizer on the area. She became agitated and indicated that she couldn't breath. An ambulance was called. Paramedics arrived and noted her to be agitated and anxious but breathing well without any wheezing. Her oxygen saturation was 100% in room air by pulse oximetry. She was transported to the ED.

Past medical history is negative. The family history is noncontributory, and social history indicates that she is a visitor to the area.

Examination reveals the following vital signs: oral temperature 36.1°C, pulse 105 beats/min, respiration 25 breaths/min, blood pressure 115/80 mm Hg, and oxygen saturation 100% in room air. She is alert, active, anxious, and cooperative. She is visibly hyperventilating and says that her hands and toes feel tingly. Eyes, ears, and mouth are normal. Pink streaking is visible over her left neck, shoulder, and anterior chest, corresponding to the areas of pain. Heartbeat is regular. Lungs are clear. Overall color and perfusion are good.

Discussion

Differential Diagnosis
- Jellyfish sting

Evaluation
She is breathing deeply and slightly fast. She is assured that her breathing is fine and when told to slow down her breathing, she does so and her anxiety level decreases, as does the tingling feeling in her hands and feet. In this geographic area, the jellyfish are largely benign. She is assessed as having a painful jellyfish sting without a significant hypersensitivity reaction.

Treatment
Oral analgesics are optional. She is placed in a hot water shower while sitting in a chair, and she states that there is immediate pain relief. She continues to remain in the hot water shower for 25 minutes, at which point she says she feels much better.

The pain has largely resolved and she has no difficulty breathing or paresthesia. Her vital signs are normal and she is discharged from the ED.

Keep in Mind
Depending on the geographic area, jellyfish might be simply painful, or highly deadly with the potential for neurologic or cardiovascular deterioration.

Jellyfish stings are typical of marine envenomations. Most toxic marine animals use toxins to disable prey for carnivorous consumption. Most of these toxins are neurotoxic proteins and are painful but incapable of inflicting death or disability in humans. However, some marine toxins are notably dangerous to humans. These generally have known geographic risk areas. Examples of these include envenomation from the Australian box jellyfish, Japanese Irukandji jellyfish, Australian blue-ringed octopus, stonefish, lionfish, and some cone shell mollusks.

The terms *box jellyfish* and *Portuguese man-of-war* are used loosely; however, these terms are not reliable in determining whether an exposure is significantly toxic. For example, the sting from the Australian box jellyfish *(Chironex fleckeri)* is highly lethal to humans, while the sting from the Hawaiian box jellyfish *(Carybdea alata)* is painful but not lethal. Portuguese man-of-war usually refers to *Physalia physalis,* also called blue bottles because they are blue in color and float on the surface of the ocean with a clear blue-tinted balloon that keeps them afloat while dangling blue tentacles below. However, the Portuguese man-of-war can refer to small blue bottles 4 cm wide or to blue bottles up to 30 cm wide, and in other instances, this term refers to a totally different jellyfish.

Jellyfish treatment recommendations are heterogeneous and largely unproven in randomized trials. For minor jellyfish stings, all improve and virtually all treatments appear to work. Because jellyfish toxin and most marine toxins are proteins, they can be hydrolyzed by proteolytic enzymes and their bioactivity can be reduced by modifying the pH or temperature of the protein. These factors form the basis for most currently recommended treatments.

Some meat tenderizer products contain papain, a proteolytic enzyme. In theory, papain should be able to hydrolyze the protein toxin into individual amino acids, neutralizing the toxin. However, the papain must be able to penetrate jellyfish tentacle stinging units (nematocysts) or penetrate the skin (toxin already injected into the skin) for toxin neutralization to take place. Unfortunately, it is not likely that such a powder can penetrate the skin or nematocysts to be effective. Additionally, only some meat tenderizer products contain papain. Some meat tenderizers are composed principally of monosodium glutamate, which has no proteolytic potential. Fresh papaya contains large amounts of papain; however, a papaya slurry is similarly unable to penetrate the skin.

Vinegar can be applied to alter the pH of the protein toxin. In theory, this should reduce the bioactivity of the protein toxin by altering its 3-dimensional configuration. However, for this to occur, the vinegar must be able to penetrate the nematocysts to neutralize the stinging units, or penetrate the skin to neutralize toxin already in the skin. Unfortunately, vinegar cannot penetrate the skin.

Heat can also denature a toxin. Marine toxins are optimized for cold temperatures. Even Hawaiian waters are relatively cold compared with body temperature. A toxin optimized for 18°C does not function well at 40°C. Unlike papain and vinegar, heat penetrates the skin well. It also penetrates nearby nematocysts.

Jellyfish stings are often treated with meat tenderizer and vinegar, but these have not been demonstrated to be effective compared to placebo. There is great controversy over whether to cleanse the skin with saline, ocean water, or freshwater, involving theoretical arguments about which of these is least likely to trigger the firing of remaining nematocysts. However, all of these recommendations are anecdotal. Hot water treatment (40°C) is better than papain and vinegar in pain reduction and visible cutaneous reaction severity. On immersion in hot water, there is nearly instant pain relief and no increase in pain resulting from additional nematocyst discharges. There is no difference in using freshwater or seawater to wash the skin. Cold packs do not relieve pain significantly because the pain recurs as soon as the cold pack is removed.

Although the treatment described here cannot be extrapolated to other marine envenomations, there are likely to be similarities because most marine toxins are proteins optimized for colder temperatures. However, serious marine envenomations such as Australian box jellyfish and Japanese Irukandji jellyfish stings require advanced life support and cannot be treated with hot water alone.

Recommended Reading

Nomura JT, Sato RL, Ahern RM, Snow JL, Kuwaye TT, Yamamoto LG. A randomized paired comparison trial of cutaneous treatments for acute jellyfish *(Carybdea alata)* stings. *Am J Emerg Med.* 2002;20:624–626

Thomas CS, Scott SA, Galanis DJ, Goto RS. Box jellyfish *(Carybdea alata)* in Waikiki. The analgesic effect of sting-aid, Adolph's meat tenderizer and fresh water on their stings: a double-blinded, randomized, placebo-controlled clinical trial. *Hawaii Med J.* 2001;60:205–210

Thomas CS, Scott SA, Galanis DJ, Goto RS. Box jellyfish *(Carybdea alata)* in Waikiki: their influx cycle plus the analgesic effect of hot and cold packs on their stings to swimmers at the beach: a randomized, placebo-controlled, clinical trial. *Hawaii Med J.* 2001;60:100–107

Chapter 32

Pool Suction Injury

Presentation

A 5-year-old boy was swimming in a hotel pool when he sat on the bottom of the pool and became firmly attached by suction to the filter cover. The patient's head was not submerged, but he was entrapped for 5 to 10 minutes until the pump could be manually disabled by a hotel employee. The suction from the filter extracted stool. He experienced some initial skin abrasion and bleeding. Now, in the emergency department (ED), the patient denies abdominal pain. His parents deny emesis. The patient is able to walk and has been acting normally since the incident occurred. He has no pain if left alone, but he experiences at least moderate discomfort when he moves his legs.

The patient is well perfused and has normal vital signs. His abdomen is soft, nontender, and nondistended with normal bowel sounds. Examination of the buttocks reveals a large circular ecchymotic zone that encompasses the inferior buttocks, ischial-perineal regions, and proximal posterior thighs, but that stops short of his posterior scrotum (Figure 32-1). There is no scrotal swelling, erythema, or tenderness. There is no penile bruising and no blood at the urethral meatus (Figure 32-2). His anus shows no visible trauma, bleeding, or prolapse.

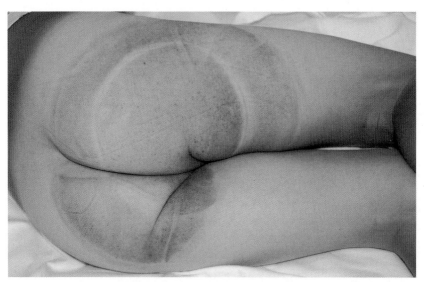

Figure 32-1

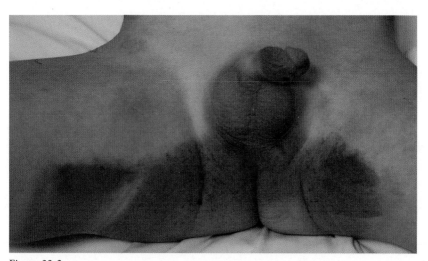

Figure 32-2

Discussion

Differential Diagnosis
- Accidental suction injury
- Inflicted injury

Evaluation
Although classic teaching in child protection is that patterned skin injuries are suspicious for abuse, these findings are entirely consistent with the mechanism described. Nothing is present during the examination that suggests a submersion event or anything else that might carry a risk of pulmonary or neurologic sequelae. Serial abdominal examinations are performed over several hours in the ED and reveal no evidence of peritoneal irritation. A urinalysis reveals only trace blood and does not suggest evidence of suction injury to the urethra.

The patient's injuries are limited to a large ecchymosis from the suction. There is no clinical evidence of any other serious gastrointestinal, genitourinary, musculoskeletal, or intraabdominal injury.

Treatment
His parents are advised to provide stool softeners, oral narcotic analgesics, and local supportive measures. You instruct them to return to the ED if the boy experiences any increased local or abdominal pain, intolerance of oral intake, difficulty with urination or defecation, rectal bleeding, or evidence of rectal prolapse. The local discomfort resolves rapidly, without abdominal or gastrointestinal symptoms.

Keep in Mind
This injury mechanism is hard to abort once it begins and usually requires interruption of the swimming pool pump. Because of this difficulty and the rapidity of onset, even vigilant adult supervision may not suffice to avoid this kind of accident. Prevention is the only true solution and includes the use of interconnected double drains, antivortex covers, and grates to prevent the formation of a tight seal with the perineum.

Although this patient's injury is limited to the skin with an uneventful recovery, more severe injuries ranging from minor prolapse to transanal or perineal evisceration may occur and may result in severe bowel injury or extensive loss. If suction pulls the victim's head below the water surface, drowning may occur.

Recommended Reading

Cain WS, Howell CG, Ziegler MM, Finley AJ, Asch MJ, Grant JP. Rectosigmoid perforation and intestinal evisceration from transanal suction. *J Pediatr Surg.* 1983;18:10–13

Centers for Disease Control and Prevention. Suction-drain injury in a public wading pool—North Carolina, 1991. *MMWR Morb Mortal Wkly Rep.* 1992;41:333–335

Gomez-Juarez M, Cascales P, Garcia-Olmo D, et al. Complete evisceration of the small intestine through a perianal wound as a result of suction at a wading pool. *J Trauma.* 2001;51:398–399

Chapter 33

Diving Into Shallow Water

Presentation

A 7-year-old boy was diving off a ledge when he landed headfirst in shallow water. He was pulled in a drowsy state from the water by lifeguards. While maintaining his airway, the lifeguards placed the patient in full cervical spine immobilization and called 911. When the patient became more alert, he complained of pain to his upper neck region. Paramedics transported the patient to the emergency department.

Your examination reveals the following vital signs: temperature 37.0°C, pulse 100 beats/min, respiration 20 breaths/min, blood pressure 125/80 mm Hg, and oxygen saturation 100% on oxygen. He is now alert, cooperative, and apprehensive. He is secured on a spine board. He complains of neck pain. He is able to move his fingers, hands, feet, and toes. Overall color and perfusion are good.

Discussion

Differential Diagnosis
- Jefferson fracture
- Cervical spine compression fracture
- Cervical strain
- Head trauma

Evaluation

You obtain a lateral neck radiograph, but no definite bony abnormalities are seen (Figure 33-1). The prevertebral soft tissue is slightly widened. This finding could be an artifact of flexion positioning (although the patient's neck is in a lordotic position) or hemorrhage from a fracture. While manually maintaining cervical spine immobilization, an open-mouth odontoid view is obtained (Figure 33-2). At first glance, this appears to be a poorly taken radiograph. With neck pain and manual cervical spine stabilization, this view is not easily obtained. However, even in a radiograph such as

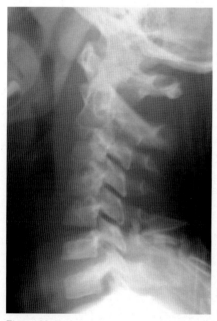

this, you still note some important features. The lateral margins of the lateral masses of C1 are sufficiently visible to identify whether a Jefferson fracture is present. The Jefferson fracture is a bursting fracture of the ring of C1.

Figure 33-3 outlines the important structures from the original radiograph (LM indicates lateral masses, which are the outer aspects of the ring of C1). If the ring of C1 is burst open, the lateral masses are displaced outward. The outlined structure below the lateral masses are the lateral aspects of C2. The lateral masses should be

Figure 33-1

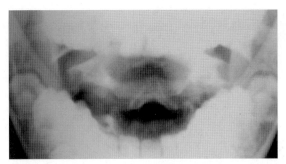

Figure 33-2

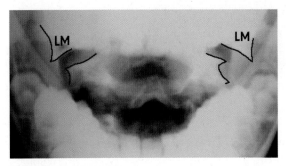

Figure 33-3

approximately aligned with the lateral aspects of C2. In this case, the lateral masses of C1 are clearly displaced outward, relative to the lateral aspects of C2. This is highly suggestive that the ring of C1 has burst open, and you diagnose a Jefferson fracture.

Treatment

The patient is maintained in cervical spine immobilization. A computed tomography (CT) scan of the cervical spine is obtained (Figure 33-4), and it confirms a Jefferson fracture. A spine surgeon is consulted. The patient's upper and lower extremity function continues to remain normal.

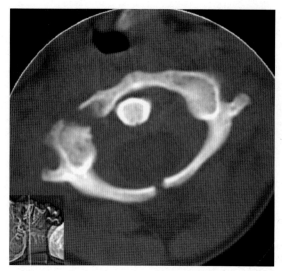

Figure 33-4

Keep in Mind

The Jefferson fracture (bursting fracture of C1) occurs with axial loading, or a force applied along the long axis of the neck. Examples of this would be diving headfirst into shallow water, as in this case, or a football player driving his helmet into the goalpost. These are both classic mechanisms for the Jefferson fracture. As the cervical spine is compressed, C2 pushes into the center of C1, bursting open the ring of C1.

In the CT image of the ring of C1 in Figure 33-4, a fracture is clearly visible. The odontoid (dens) and the spinal cord are visible within the ring. A general principle of a rigid ring is that when it breaks, it always breaks in 2 places. Imagine a hard pretzel ring and breaking it. It is almost impossible to break the pretzel in only one place. This principle applies to the ring of C1 as well. In nearly all instances, the ring fractures in 2 places. Because only one fracture is visible, the other fracture must be through the growth plate at the posterior aspect of the ring (the open section of the ring). A transverse ligament separates the odontoid from the spinal cord. In some cases, the transverse ligament ruptures, resulting in additional instability and increasing the risk of spinal cord injury.

The images in figures 33-5 and 33-6 are from the same patient. The odontoid view is much clearer. Figure 33-6 outlines the lateral masses of C1 and the outer aspect of C2 below it. Again, the lateral masses are displaced outward. Although this view is of better quality, the Jefferson fracture was still visible on the initial view.

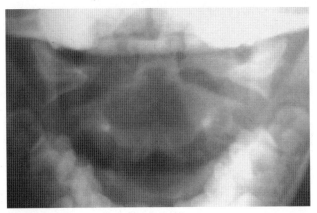

Figure 33-5

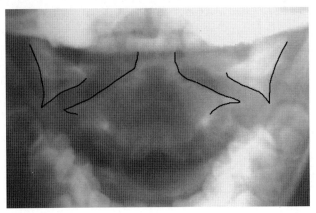

Figure 33-6

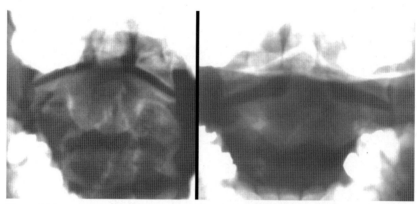

Figure 33-7

The images in Figure 33-7 are odontoid views from different patients who do not have a Jefferson fracture. In these cases, the lateral masses are nearly perfectly aligned with the lateral aspects of C2 below it.

Recommended Reading

Yee LL. The Jefferson fracture. In: Yamamoto LG, Inaba AS, DiMauro R, eds. *Radiology Cases in Pediatric Emergency Medicine.* Vol 5, case 4. October 1996. Available at: http://www.hawaii.edu/medicine/pediatrics/ pemxray/v5c04.html. Accessed December 17, 2008

Chapter 34

Pedestrian and Motor Vehicle Collision

Presentation

A 10-year-old boy was rollerblading in a parking garage (Figure 34-1). A van sped around the corner and struck him, then partially rolled forward over him as the car tried to stop. A bystander called 911. The boy was initially crying in pain without any loss of consciousness. Ambulance personnel arrived in about 20 minutes and noted the boy to be lethargic. His head and neck were immobilized on a spine board at the scene. Intravenous (IV) normal saline was started in transit, infusing rapidly. Blow-by oxygen was delivered. He was breathing spontaneously. Radio communication to the emergency department (ED) reported his vital signs to be pulse 180 beats/min, respiration 30 breaths/min, blood pressure 60 mm Hg systolic. Electrocardiographic monitoring showed sinus tachycardia. The emergency responders noted many abrasions and contusions as well as a thigh deformity. Estimated time of arrival to your ED is 8 minutes.

When you examine the boy at arrival, he is essentially the same. His blood pressure is 65/40 mm Hg. Oxygen saturation is 100% on supplemental oxygen. He is breathing spontaneously. His legs are secured on the spine board in such a way that the thigh deformity is not very obvious.

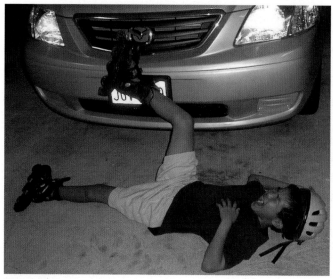

Figure 34-1

Discussion

Differential Diagnosis
- Hemorrhagic shock
- Abdominal hemorrhage
- Femur fracture

Evaluation
Although laboratory evaluation and imaging studies may be ordered, the patient was hypotensive in the field and remains hypotensive in the ED; therefore, resuscitation should take priority.

Trauma resuscitation is beyond the scope of this single case presentation; however, a general ABCDE approach should be followed.

- *Airway.* The boy is currently breathing on his own. It is not clear whether he needs to be intubated. If there is any further pulmonary or cardiac deterioration, he should be intubated orally using a paralyzing drug such as rocuronium. A sedative might greatly worsen his cardiovascular status, so the benefit of a sedative must be evaluated carefully.

- *Breathing.* He is currently breathing on his own and his oxygen saturation is 100% on supplemental oxygen. Air exchange can be assessed by auscultation.
- *Circulation.* He is hypotensive, most likely as a result of hemorrhagic shock. Crystalloid infusion alone is likely to be insufficient. It will take at least 15 to 30 minutes to obtain type and cross-matched blood. In the meantime, O-negative packed red blood cells should be infused as soon as he arrives. Hypotension can also be caused by a tension pneumothorax, but his status is not deteriorating rapidly, his oxygenation is maintained, and his breathing pattern is normal.
- *Disability.* His neurologic function should be assessed quickly. He can move his hands, fingers, feet, and toes. He complains of pain in his left thigh. He is able to speak and can answer your questions. A lateral neck radiograph is obtained.
- *Exposure.* His clothes should be removed so that all injuries are visible. At some point, his back should be examined without compromising spine immobilization.

Treatment

O-negative blood is warmed and ready for infusion on arrival of the patient, so IV access must be obtained immediately. In this case, an IV line has already been started. If there is any delay in obtaining IV access, an intraosseous infusion site should be used for volume expansion until an IV can be started. A surgeon should be called. The patient should be prepared for a computed tomography (CT) scan.

If the patient is conscious and uncomfortable, analgesics can be administered to make the patient more comfortable. Intravenous narcotic analgesics can worsen hypotension, so its benefits must be weighed against its adverse effects.

Keep in Mind

The pediatric heart is very healthy. As circulatory volume is lost, the heart can increase cardiac output by increasing its rate and stroke volume. Thus, blood pressure can be maintained during the phase of early shock. Once hypotension is present, the patient is in a more advanced and serious stage of shock. Approximately 25% of the blood volume or more has been lost by the time hypotension has developed. Although infusing crystalloid while monitoring for improvement is commonly recommended, a general rule of thumb is that 3 mL of crystalloid is required to replace 1 mL of blood loss. Hypotension recognized early after a traumatic injury suggests rapid blood loss, which implies that crystalloid alone is likely to be insufficient to volume resuscitate the patient. Late shock has a poorer prognosis than early shock; thus, treating shock aggressively to prevent worsening to a more severe degree is beneficial.

Because blood takes 15 to 30 minutes or more to type and cross-match, O-negative packed red blood cells should be infused while the cross-match is taking place. Although it is difficult to reduce the total time required for the cross-matching process, even if it is given top priority in the blood bank, the urgency of the cross-match request must be communicated clearly to the laboratory, perhaps by having a nurse or resident from the ED present in the blood bank while the cross-match is being performed. Additionally, for EDs that do not transfuse blood frequently, further delays may occur. Blood transfusion requires special equipment such as filters, IV tubing, blood warmers, identification banding, and labels. Required safety precautions and acquiring equipment can delay the transfusion, especially if nursing personnel are not familiar with this process.

A CT scan is the quickest way to assess the brain, abdomen, and pelvis. Computed tomography scanners can now scan the head, neck, and torso in a few seconds. This gives emergency physicians a tremendous diagnostic advantage in assessing the patient's status. The chest can still be quickly and accurately evaluated by conventional chest radiograph, but once the patient is in the CT scanner, a head-to-pelvis scan can be faster, although the x-ray exposure dose is substantially higher, and if the patient is moved out of the ED, the intensity of patient monitoring and the ability to resuscitate the patient is less robust.

Recommended Reading

Tepas JJ, Fallat ME, Moriarty TM. Trauma. In: Gausche-Hill M, Fuchs S, Yamamoto L, eds. *APLS: The Pediatric Emergency Medicine Resource.* 4th rev ed. Sudbury, MA: Jones and Bartlett Publishers; 2007:268–323

Chapter 35

Rollover Motor Vehicle Collision Causing Severe Abdominal and Back Pain

Presentation

A 5-year-old girl arrives by ambulance after being involved in a high-speed motor vehicle collision while seated on a relative's lap with a lap and shoulder belt fastened over both passengers. Other vehicle occupants experienced serious injuries and have been transported to adult trauma centers. Your patient complains primarily of abdominal and back pain. Interventions during transport included spinal immobilization and insertion of an intravenous line, but no resuscitative measures were required. She has experienced no loss of consciousness or respiratory distress, and she denies paresthesias, weakness, or pain to the head, neck, chest, and extremities.

She is tachycardic (140 beats/min) and slightly pale, but otherwise well perfused with normal vital signs including blood pressure 115/78 mm Hg. She has a horizontal bruise across her midabdomen (Figure 35-1) with diffuse tenderness. A wide region of swelling and tenderness overlies the midlumbar spine. She has normal distal strength and normal distal and perianal sensation.

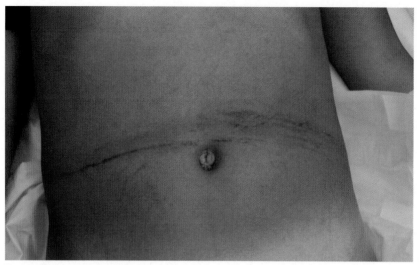

Figure 35-1

Discussion

Differential Diagnosis

- Blunt trauma due to seat belt–related injury
- Axial skeletal injury
- Intraabdominal solid or hollow organ injury

Evaluation

Given the obviously serious mechanism of injury, the diagnosis of blunt trauma is not in question. Her pallor and mild tachycardia raise concern for occult blood loss, and the location of the findings suggest intraabdominal injury and lumbar fracture.

Screening trauma laboratory results include hemoglobin 11.0 g/dL, alanine aminotransferase 35 U/L, and amylase 45 U/L. Plain radiographs of the lumbar spine reveal no obvious fracture; however, anterior widening between L4 and L5 is evident on the lateral view (Figure 35-2). She undergoes computed tomography (CT) imaging of the abdomen and lumbar spine and is then admitted to a monitored unit.

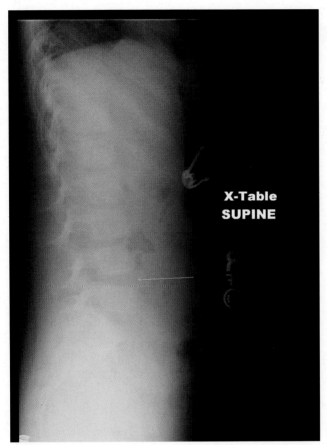

**X-Table
SUPINE**

Figure 35-2

Treatment

Initial CT scan demonstrates a small amount of free fluid within the pelvis but no solid organ injury and no free air. The L4 vertebral body has anterior wedging, and the L4-L5 disk space is widened anteriorly with widening of the space between the L3 and L4 spinous processes (Figure 35-3). Overnight, she experiences increasing abdominal pain, and follow-up CT imaging reveals increased intraperitoneal fluid with dilated proximal small bowel and a transition to normal caliber bowel distally. She therefore undergoes exploratory laparotomy with resection of an ileal perforation (figures 35-4 and 35-5) with primary anastomosis.

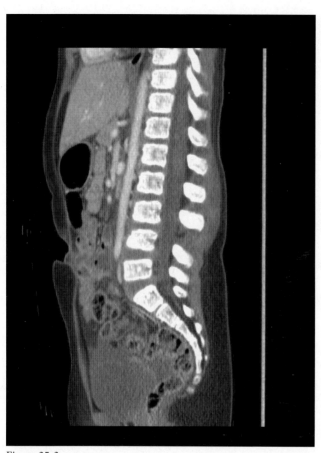

Figure 35-3

After recovery from her laparotomy, her lumbar injury is evaluated. Magnetic resonance imaging demonstrates evidence of a ligamentous injury between the L3 and L4 spinous processes without compromise of the cord or canal. She subsequently undergoes posterior fusion of L3-L4. After surgery, she experiences progressively improved mobility with the use of an orthotic device and oral analgesics.

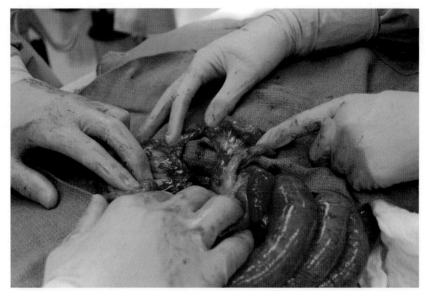

Figure 35-4

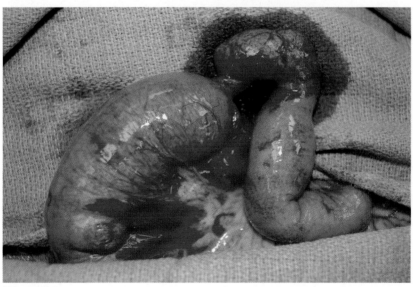

Figure 35-5

Courtesy of Nicholas Saenz, MD

Keep in Mind

Seat belts, particularly when applied incorrectly, produce a predictable pattern of injuries. Rapid deceleration against a lap belt can cause bowel, solid organ, and mesenteric injuries. The seat belt acts as a fulcrum in a flexion-distraction mechanism, resulting in bony or ligamentous injury to the lumbar spine (the Chance fracture). Inadequate torso restraint allows the head to strike against the interior of the vehicle.

Suboptimal restraint confers a 3- to 4-fold increased risk for intraabdominal injury, particularly to the hollow viscera. Children in the 4- to 8-year age range are at particularly high risk for poor restraint and thus experience higher rates of abdominal injury. Many are graduated from car safety seats or belt-positioning booster seats too soon, resulting in placement of the lap belt over the abdomen rather than the pelvis. The shoulder belt rides high, and the child often places the belt under the arm or behind the back.

Even at relatively low speeds, improperly restrained children may experience substantial seat belt–related injury. Several distinct mechanisms are described. *Submarining* begins with a lap belt in its proper position around the pelvis, and the collision causes the pelvis to slide under the belt. With *presubmarining*, the belt is already positioned improperly over the abdomen. *Jackknifing* of the torso over the belt may complicate submarining or presubmarining. The child sharing a seat belt with an adult experiences the deceleration force of the adult's larger body against the restraint.

Even if the adequacy of restraint is unknown, children with a seat belt sign have 3 times' greater risk of an intraabdominal injury than those without. The increased risk is particularly a result of intestinal and pancreatic injuries. The combination of lap belt contusion with abdominal and lumbar pain should raise suspicion for a combination of serious abdominal and skeletal injuries. Abdominal imaging is warranted but may be deceptively normal at the outset, mandating continued clinical vigilance with serial examinations and repeated imaging, as well as surgical exploration if tenderness persists or increases.

Recommended Reading

American Academy of Pediatrics, Committee on Injury and Poison Prevention. Selecting and using the most appropriate car safety seats for growing children: guidelines for counseling parents. *Pediatrics.* 2002;109:550–553

Arbogast KB, Kent RW, Menon RA, Ghati Y, Durbin DR, Rouhana SW. Mechanisms of abdominal organ injury in seat belt–restrained children. *J Trauma.* 2007;62:1473–1480

Durbin DR, Arbogast KB, Moll EK. Seat belt syndrome in children: a case report and review of the literature. *Pediatr Emerg Care.* 2001;17:474–477

Nance ML, Lutz N, Arbogast KB, et al. Optimal restraint reduces the risk of abdominal injury in children involved in motor vehicle crashes. *Ann Surg.* 2004;239:127–131

Sokolove PE, Kuppermann N, Holmes JF. Association between the "seat belt sign" and intra-abdominal injury in children with blunt torso trauma. *Acad Emerg Med.* 2005;12:808–813

Chapter 36

Unrestrained Occupant in Motor Vehicle Collision Presenting With Chest and Abdominal Pain

Presentation

A 9-year-old girl was an unrestrained backseat passenger in a vehicle involved in a head-on collision. She was thrown against the car's console and developed pain to the chest, head, and abdomen, particularly on the left side. There has been no loss of consciousness, respiratory distress, vomiting, seizures, or visible bleeding. She is transported with an intravenous line and spinal immobilization. She receives no other interventions and is described by paramedics as having been stable en route.

Her vital signs at arrival are as follows: temperature 36.7°C, pulse 84 beats/min, respiration 24 breaths/min, blood pressure 125/62 mm Hg, and room air oxyhemoglobin saturation 100%. The primary survey is normal; her Glasgow Coma Scale score is 15. The secondary survey reveals no obvious trauma to the face, scalp, or neck. She has tenderness and an abrasion over the left lower ribs anteriorly without chest wall instability. Abdominal examination reveals decreased bowel sounds with tenderness on the left. The pelvis is stable, and extremities have no tenderness or deformity. There is no evidence of anogenital bleeding or trauma.

Discussion

Differential Diagnosis
- Isolated chest or abdominal wall contusion
- Rib fracture
- Intrathoracic trauma (eg, pulmonary contusion, pneumothorax)
- Intraabdominal trauma, including injury to spleen, kidney, adrenal gland, or pancreas

Evaluation
Initial trauma laboratory results include the following: white blood cells 12,100/μL, hemoglobin 12.1 g/dL, hematocrit 36.3%, alanine aminotransferase 25 U/L, and amylase 36 U/L. Radiographs of cervical spine and chest reveal no fractures, dislocation, or pneumothorax.

Treatment
The patient is hemodynamically normal on presentation; during transport and at the emergency department (ED), she requires no resuscitative measures. However, there is clinical evidence to suggest an intraabdominal solid organ injury, lung contusion, or both. Intravenous contrast enhanced computed tomography imaging of the abdomen and pelvis demonstrates a splenic laceration (Figure 36-1) with evidence of ongoing extravasation in the upper pole (Figure 36-2).

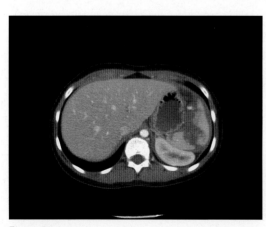

Figure 36-1

Over the next several hours, the patient becomes tachycardic, and despite transfusion of packed red blood cells, her blood pressure decreases to 88/42 mm Hg and her hemoglobin falls to 9.5 g/dL. She undergoes

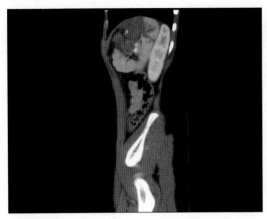

Figure 36-2

embolization of a splenic arterial branch. Her subsequent inpatient course while on strict bed rest is unremarkable; there is no further evidence of blood loss or hemodynamic instability.

Her hemoglobin is normal and stable at the time of discharge. She is counseled to avoid strenuous physical activity or contact sports for 6 weeks.

Keep in Mind

Absence of major external injury or rib fracture does not imply absence of serious solid organ injury.

Trauma laboratory evaluation may have poor sensitivity for splenic injury, and clinical examination and ED course should dictate the decision to proceed with imaging.

Nonoperative management of solid organ injury has become standard practice in the management of pediatric blunt abdominal trauma. Although contrast blush or extravasation is controversial as a predictor of failure of nonoperative management in hepatic or splenic injury, ongoing hemodynamic instability or laboratory measures of ongoing blood loss despite blood replacement are important indicators for more aggressive intervention. The decision to proceed with operative management is tempered by the risk of postsplenectomy sepsis.

Recommended Reading

Stylianos S, Pearl RH. Abdominal trauma. In: Grosfeld JL, O'Neill JA, Coran AG, Fonkalsrud EW, Caldamone AA, eds. *Pediatric Surgery.* 6th ed. Philadelphia, PA: CV Mosby; 2006:295–316

Chapter 37

Motor Vehicle Collision and Sudden Deterioration Following Intubation

Presentation

A 2-year-old girl is sitting unrestrained in the front seat of a car that hits a telephone pole head-on at about 40 mph. Driver and front passenger air bags deployed. The driver is conscious and complains of mild chest tenderness. When the ambulance arrives, emergency personnel find the child unconscious, blue, and apneic. Her heart rate is 80 beats/min. She is immediately intubated. Her color improves, and her heart rate is now 160 beats/min. Many bruises and abrasions are evident over her trunk and head. Transport time to the emergency department (ED) is 5 minutes. The ambulance team transports the patient immediately and communicates with the ED while in transport. An intravenous (IV) line could not be started during transport.

When you examine her on her arrival at the ED, you note the following vital signs: pulse 170 beats/min, blood pressure 70/35 mm Hg, respiration 50 breaths/min (manually ventilated), and oxygen saturation 100% on oxygen (via the endotracheal tube). She is not responsive to painful or verbal stimuli. There are multiple abrasions over her face, forehead and scalp; hematomas, abrasions and bruises over her chest; and superficial abrasions over her extremities. Pupils are equal and reactive. No blood is visible in the ear canals, tympanic membranes, or nose. She is on a spine board with her neck partially immobilized. Her heartbeat is regular, and her breath sounds are clear and equal. Her abdomen is soft with active bowel sounds.

An IV line is started and normal saline is infused at a rapid rate. Blood studies including a type and cross-match are ordered. O-negative packed red blood cells are infusing. While you are proceeding with her evaluation and treatment, her color deteriorates rapidly. Heart rate drops to

50 beats/min, and blood pressure is 30/15 mm Hg. The patient's breath sounds are diminished bilaterally, but are more diminished on the left.

Discussion

Differential Diagnosis
• Tension pneumothorax

Evaluation
Sudden cardiorespiratory deterioration such as this suggests the presence of a tension pneumothorax or a pneumopericardium or tamponade. Tension pneumothorax is far more common. With vital signs such as heart rate 50 beats/min and blood pressure 30/15 mm Hg, you cannot wait to confirm the diagnosis by chest radiograph.

Treatment
Immediate action is required. You perform needle thoracentesis in the left hemithorax followed by a tube thoracostomy, and the patient's oxygenation and circulatory parameters improve dramatically.

Keep in Mind
In a tension pneumothorax, one lung has collapsed and air is trapped in the affected hemithorax. This air trapping compresses the collapsed lung, the contralateral lung, and the heart. This phenomenon rapidly worsens as the tensioning air pressure in the affected hemithorax increases, resulting in severe hypoxia (refractory to increases in inspired oxygen) and hypotension. Death will result shortly unless the tension is relieved immediately.

A nontension pneumothorax results in a collapse or partial collapse of the affected lung. Although this usually results in dyspnea and chest pain, it does not cause sudden respiratory and cardiovascular collapse. A nontension pneumothorax can be confirmed on a chest radiograph to assess the need for treatment. However, a tension pneumothorax is a true emergency that requires immediate treatment.

Figure 37-1 shows the rapid progression of a tension pneumothorax. A tension pneumothorax most often occurs in 2 clinical situations, positive pressure ventilation and penetrating chest wound.

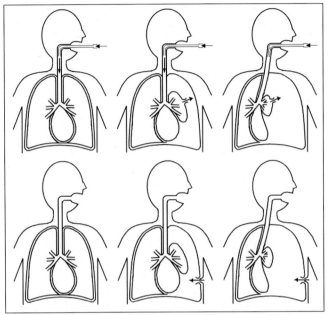

Figure 37-1

In the top images in Figure 37-1, a ventilator is pushing air into the lungs via an endotracheal tube. When an air leak in the left lung occurs, the left lung partially collapses. During the exhalation phase, the air leak seals, forming a one-way valve that opens with each positive pressure breath from the ventilator and closes during each exhalation phase. With each ventilator cycle, more air is trapped in the left hemithorax. Not only does this further collapse the affected lung, but it also compresses the contralateral lung and the heart, which results in rapidly progressive hypoxia and hypotension.

In the bottom images in Figure 37-1, a penetrating chest wound has caused an air leak into the pleural space and the left lung partially collapses. When the patient inhales, the chest expands, creating negative pressure in the pleural space. More air is sucked into the left side of the chest. During exhalation, the chest wall seals the air leak, forming a one-way valve that opens with each inhalation (chest wall expansion) and closes during each exhalation. With each breath, more air is trapped in the left hemithorax.

The result is the same—the affected lung further collapses, and the contra-lateral lung and the heart are compressed, resulting in rapidly progressive hypoxia and hypotension.

Needle thoracentesis is the most commonly recommended rapid method of decompressing the affected hemithorax. Although this procedure does not expand the affected lung, it does relieve the compression on the contralateral lung and the heart to relieve the hypoxia and hypotension.

It may be hard to determine which side the pneumothorax is on. Auscultation is difficult because the good lung is compressed and not aerating. You can attempt to assess whether tracheal deviation is present. The trachea deviates away from the side of the pneumothorax. If a penetrating chest wound is present, the pneumothorax is most likely on that side. If you cannot determine which side is affected, the thoracentesis should be attempted on any side, and if not successful, then attempted on the other side.

The procedure is as follows. Attach a needle or a stiff wall IV catheter to a large syringe (50–60 mL). The plunger on the syringe should be at 0 mL. Insert the needle into the apex or the lateral aspect of the suspected hemithorax. Although a particular rib interspace is often specified, it is hard to count ribs during a true emergency. Note that the target is large. Visualize the apex of the pleural cavity or enter the chest laterally. Entering the air-filled hemithorax can be done from nearly any position in the chest, but the apex is best. If possible, advance the needle over a rib (as close as possible to the superior surface of the rib), rather than under the rib, because the intercostal neurovascular bundle travels under each rib. As the needle is advanced into the chest, apply negative pressure to the syringe. When the needle tip enters the pneumothorax cavity, a large gush of air will be appreciated in the aspirating syringe. Aspirate as much as possible, then remove the syringe from the needle, empty the syringe, reattach the syringe, and aspirate again. Continue to do this repeatedly. The patient's oxygenation and circulation should improve because this procedure should relieve pressure on the heart and the contralateral lung. If no gush of air is felt, attempt the same procedure on the other side. Although a stopcock may be attached between the needle and syringe to prevent more air from entering the chest when the syringe is removed, this is not necessary for a tension pneumothorax. In a tension pneumothorax, air will only flow out because it is under pressure. The stopcock can make it harder to continuously aspirate the chest.

While someone is aspirating the chest continuously to stabilize the patient, another person must set up to perform a tube thoracostomy. Identify the anterior axillary line adjacent to the nipple. This is the chest tube entry point. If the needle thoracentesis is placed in the apex of the chest, the chest tube entry point should be easily accessible. Placing the needle thoracentesis in the lateral chest will interfere with the placement of the chest tube.

Infiltrate lidocaine into the chest tube entry point site. Make an incision parallel to the ribs. Using a mosquito hemostat, penetrate this incision and bluntly advance the instrument over a rib (instead of under a rib) until it advances into the hemithorax. Advance the chest tube into the tunnel without the trocar. Although the tube may be advanced with a trocar, the tip of the metal trocar can puncture the aorta, vena cava, heart, or other large vessels if it is advanced too far. It is safer to advance the tube without the trocar. Point the tube in the superior direction. Suture the tube in place. Continuous low-level suction can be applied to the tube to reexpand the affected lung. The needle thoracentesis aspiration can be stopped to see if the patient's cardiopulmonary status remains stable. If so, the thoracentesis needle can be removed.

Recommended Reading

King BR, King C, Coates WC. Critical procedures. Section 15. Thoracic procedures. In: Gausche-Hill M, Fuchs S, Yamamoto L, eds. *APLS: The Pediatric Emergency Medicine Resource*. 4th rev ed. Sudbury, MA: Jones and Bartlett Publishers; 2007:741–746

Tepas JJ, Fallat ME, Moriarty TM. Trauma. In: Gausche-Hill M, Fuchs S, Yamamoto L, eds. *APLS: The Pediatric Emergency Medicine Resource*. 4th rev ed. Sudbury, MA: Jones and Bartlett Publishers; 2007:268–323

Part 5

Central Nervous System Presentations

Lethargic Infant

Presentation

An 8-month-old boy was assessed by his primary care physician 2 days ago for a presumed viral illness. He is now brought to the emergency department by his mother because he seems sleepy, weak, and lethargic. He has had fever for 5 days to 38.3°C, decreased appetite, decreased activity, and occasional clear emesis. Because the child has appeared fairly well, his mother was not alarmed because these symptoms (except for lethargy) occurred in her other children. However, this evening, she notes that her son is more lethargic than before.

Past medical, social, and family histories are not contributory.

Examination of vital signs reveals the following: rectal temperature 39.1°C, pulse 120 beats/min, respiration 30 breaths/min, blood pressure 70/45 mm Hg, and oxygen saturation 98% in room air.

The infant appears well nourished and he is in no distress, although he is lethargic. He does not move much and he does not respond to painful stimuli. Examination of head, eyes, ears, nose, and throat reveal nothing abnormal. The patient's mucous membranes are moist. His neck is supple, his heartbeat regular, and his lungs clear. His abdomen is flat and soft with active bowel sounds. His muscle tone is decreased. Deep tendon reflexes are 2+. Color and perfusion are good.

Discussion

Differential Diagnosis
- Coma
- Drug ingestion (sedative)
- Hypoglycemia
- Diabetic ketoacidosis
- Seizure not witnessed
- Meningitis
- Intussusception
- Infant botulism
- Guillain-Barré syndrome

Evaluation
A bedside glucose is 25 mg/dL. While other blood samples are collected for testing, he is treated with IV glucose. The patient's complete blood count is normal. His glucose level is 25 mg/dL, sodium is 131 mmol/L, potassium is 3.3 mmol/L, chloride is 98 mmol/L, and bicarbonate is 18 mmol/L. Urinalysis specific gravity is 1.022, ketones are moderate, and there are 0 to 1 white blood cells per high-power field.

Other actions that could be considered in this case include lumbar puncture and empiric antibiotics if sepsis or meningitis is suspected. Given the extremely low glucose level, a blood sample should be drawn for metabolic studies before glucose correction if possible.

Treatment
The child was diagnosed with ketotic hypoglycemia. He was immediately treated with intravenous (IV) glucose, resulting in improved activity and responsiveness. Intravenous naloxone is reasonable as a trial even if a drug overdose is not suspected.

Keep in Mind
Hypoglycemia is more common in infants and young children with limited caloric and nutritional reserves. Some hypoglycemic infants and children have minor metabolic disorders, although other metabolic disorders can be

serious. Gluconeogenesis should generally occur in starvation states to prevent hypoglycemia. If this process if defective, insufficient, or not regulated sufficiently, hypoglycemia can result.

Ketosis occurs in most patients with hypoglycemia because fat is metabolized as an alternate energy substrate. Ketotic hypoglycemia is not a metabolic diagnosis, but rather the expected occurrence of ketosis with hypoglycemia. Marked hypoglycemia without ketosis is suggestive of pathologic processes such as fatty acid oxidative metabolic disorders. Thus, the absence of ketosis should be more alarming than the presence of ketosis in a hypoglycemic state. Ketosis is most easily identified by urine dipstick testing. This can be a useful screening test for patients with hypoglycemia to screen for a metabolic defect.

If a metabolic disorder is suspected, it is useful to draw a blood sample before treating the hypoglycemia because the hypoglycemia state should provoke a metabolic or endocrine response. Once the hypoglycemia is corrected, it will be more difficult to establish a metabolic or endocrine diagnosis. The blood specimen should be saved for tests recommended by a metabolic specialist.

Treatment of hypoglycemia can take several forms, depending on the urgency of the hypoglycemia correction. A general rule is the so-called 50 rule. The milliliters per kilogram volume multiplied by the glucose percentage should equal 50, as shown in Table 38-1.

Glucose dosing recommendations can also be found expressed as grams per kilogram. A common recommendation is 0.5 g/kg. For example, D5W indicates 5% glucose. The percentage means grams per 100 mL,

Table 38-1. The 50 Rule

Glucose Percentage	Volume, mL/kg
50%	1
25%	2
10%	5
5%	10

so D5W contains 5 g of glucose per 100 mL. Ten milliliters of D5W contains 0.5 g of glucose. Therefore, 0.5 g/kg equals 10 mL/kg of D5W (as predicted by the 50 rule). Some clinicians suggest that only half this amount be administered.

If clinical factors suggest that the hypoglycemia will persist (eg, lack of caloric intake, an overdose of insulin or an oral hypoglycemia agent), a glucose infusion will be required to maintain blood glucose and to replenish glycogen stores.

Overly aggressive glucose administration can result in hyperglycemia, which is usually harmless if transient; however, because glucose is a significant osmotic agent, large fluctuations of glucose, from low to high, could also lead to fluid shifts, some of which could be potentially harmful.

The commonly used rapid infusion volume of 20 mL/kg is twice the recommended glucose dose if the infusion volume contains 5% dextrose. Thus, administering a bolus of 20 mL/kg of 5% dextrose solutions (eg, D5NS, D5LR) is likely to result in hyperglycemia; 5% glucose is equal to 5,000 mg/dL, which can easily overwhelm the normal blood glucose of roughly 100 mg/dL if infused too fast and for too long.

Recommended Reading

Agus MS. Endocrine emergencies. In: Fleisher GR, Ludwig S, Henretig FM, Ruddy RM, Silverman BK, eds. *Textbook of Pediatric Emergency Medicine.* 5th ed. Philadelphia, PA: Lippincott Williams & Wilkins; 2006:1167–1192

Glaser N, Enns GM, Kupperman N. Metabolic disease. In: Gausche-Hill M, Fuchs S, Yamamoto L, eds. *APLS: The Pediatric Emergency Medicine Resource.* 4th rev ed. Sudbury, MA: Jones and Bartlett Publishers; 2007:186–207

Weiner DL. Metabolic emergencies. In: Fleisher GR, Ludwig S, Henretig FM, Ruddy RM, Silverman BK, eds. *Textbook of Pediatric Emergency Medicine.* 5th ed. Philadelphia, PA: Lippincott Williams & Wilkins; 2006:1193–1206

Chapter 39

Lethargy and Weakness

Presentation

A 3-year-old girl is brought to the emergency department (ED) because of lethargy and weakness. Since yesterday, she has not been very active, and her parents have noted her to be weak. She has no vomiting, headache, fever, diarrhea, or cold symptoms. Her appetite is slightly decreased.

Your examination reveals the following vital signs: rectal temperature 37.6°C, pulse 110 beats/min, respiration 30 breaths/min, blood pressure 100/75 mm Hg, and oxygen saturation 99% in room air. Her weight is at the 50th percentile. She is alert and moves about fairly well on the examination table, in no distress. She prefers not to walk. She responds well verbally. Examination of head, eyes, ears, nose, and throat is normal. Her neck is supple. Her heartbeat is regular with no murmur. Her lungs are clear with good aeration. Her abdomen is soft and nontender. Her strength is weak in all 4 extremities. Deep tendon reflexes are 1+ in her upper extremities and absent in her lower extremities.

Discussion

Differential Diagnosis
- Guillain-Barré syndrome (GBS)
- Tick paralysis
- Muscle disease

Evaluation
Laboratory evaluation is performed, with the following complete blood count findings: white blood cells 12,000/µL, 30% segmented neutrophils, 45% lymphocytes, 4% eosinophils, 21% monocytes, hemoglobin 13 g/dL, hematocrit 39%, and platelet count 280,000/µL.

Lumbar puncture is performed. Analysis of the cerebrospinal fluid (CSF) reveals the following: 1 red blood cell, 1 white blood cell, 50% lymphocytes, 50% monocytes, glucose 60 mg/dL, and protein 88 mg/dL (high). Gram stain reveals no organisms.

The patient is diagnosed with Guillain-Barré syndrome.

Treatment
Guillain-Barré syndrome is generally self-limited, with good recovery in most cases. Ventilatory support is required in patients who develop respiratory failure. Motor recovery can be accelerated by inpatient treatment with intravenous gamma globulin or plasmapheresis.

Keep in Mind
Guillain-Barré syndrome is an acute demyelinating polyneuropathy that progresses (ascends) to a flaccid paralysis. Motor symptoms dominate the clinical presentation, but sensory dysfunction is often present on careful examination. Guillain-Barré syndromes are heterogeneous. The Miller-Fisher variant occurs with ophthalmoplegia as well. Guillain-Barré syndrome cases have the potential to progress to respiratory insufficiency and failure. Frequent pulmonary function assessments should be included as part of the patient's overall evaluation. The dominant clinical findings are weakness and areflexia or extreme hyporeflexia.

The pathogenesis is an autoimmune reaction against the myelin of peripheral nerves. Analysis of CSF drawn by lumbar puncture provides valuable information that supports the diagnosis of GBS. Typically, the CSF protein is high and the cell counts are normal. Symptoms are predominantly motor.

Nerve conduction studies and electromyography are generally not performed in the ED. When performed on inpatients, these studies confirm a neuropathic (as opposed to myopathic) process.

The differential diagnosis should include spinal cord conditions. Transverse myelitis will often have a CSF pleocytosis. Magnetic resonance imaging studies are often obtained to aid clinical decision-making.

Recommended Reading

Gorelick MH, Blackwell CD. Neurologic emergencies. In: Fleisher GR, Ludwig S, Henretig FM, Ruddy RM, Silverman BK, eds. *Textbook of Pediatric Emergency Medicine.* 5th ed. Philadelphia, PA: Lippincott Williams & Wilkins; 2006:759–781

Okimura JT. Guillain-Barré syndrome. In: Yamamoto LG, Inaba AS, Okamoto JK, Patronis ME, Yamashiroya VK, eds. *Case Based Pediatrics for Medical Students and Residents.* Honolulu, HI: University of Hawaii; 2004:552–554. Available at: http://www.hawaii.edu/medicine/pediatrics/pedtext. Accessed December 30, 2008

Chapter 40

Lethargy and Poor Feeding

Presentation

A 2-month-old boy is brought to the emergency department because of lethargy and poor feeding. No fever, vomiting, diarrhea, or respiratory symptoms are evident. He has not passed stool for 2 days. He is not feeding well. He doesn't refuse the bottle; he just seems to not suck very well. Urine output is good.

Examination reveals the following vital signs: rectal temperature 37.5°C, pulse 100 beats/min, respiration 30 breaths/min, blood pressure 80/45 mm Hg, and oxygen saturation 99% in room air. His weight is at the 50th percentile. He is alert and in no distress. He is not very active, but he moves all 4 extremities. Examination of head, eyes, ears, nose, and throat is normal, except that when an index finger is placed in his mouth, his suck is weak. His neck is supple. His heartbeat is regular with no murmur. Lungs are clear. His abdomen is very soft and bowel sounds are hypoactive. Genitalia are normal. Deep tendon reflexes are 1+ with noticeable hypotonia in all extremities.

Discussion

Differential Diagnosis
- Hypoglycemia
- Sepsis
- Infant botulism
- Guillain-Barré syndrome
- Muscle disease
- Other neurologic disease

Evaluation
Laboratory evaluation is performed; glucose is found to be 100 mg/dL. Complete blood count reveals the following: white blood cells 13,000/μL, 35% segmented neutrophils, 40% lymphocytes, 4% eosinophils, 21% monocytes, hemoglobin 12.5 g/dL, hematocrit 40%, and platelet count 400,000/μL.

Lumbar puncture is performed. Analysis of the cerebrospinal fluid reveals the following: 0 red blood cells, 1 white blood cell, 50% lymphocytes, 50% monocytes, glucose 60 mg/dL, and protein 12 mg/dL. Gram stain revealed no organisms.

Treatment
The patient is hospitalized, and therapy with intravenous ampicillin and gentamicin is begun to cover the possibility of sepsis. Two hours after the gentamicin is administered, the patient experiences a respiratory arrest. The patient is found apneic, hypoxic, and bradycardic. He is mask ventilated and his heart rate and oxygen saturation promptly improve. However, no respiratory effort is present, so he is intubated, placed on a ventilator, and transferred to the intensive care unit.

Infant botulism is suspected. He is ventilator-dependent for 3 weeks. A stool sample (obtained after an enema) tests positive for botulinum toxin. He is supported with mechanical ventilation and parenteral nutrition. He slowly improves and eventually recovers with good neurologic function.

Keep in Mind

Infant botulism is caused by the toxin formed by *Clostridium botulinum*, an anaerobic spore-forming organism found in soil. It can contaminate food substances. Standard canning practices eliminate spore contamination by heating (cooking) the contents of all canned foods. Although honey is often implicated in infant botulism, in most cases, honey has not been consumed. Although some samples of honey have been demonstrated to contain botulism spores, confirming that honey is a significant causal factor in the majority of infant botulism cases is difficult to ascertain. Earlier risk exposure studies noted that patients with infant botulism frequently ate honey; however, it should be noted that patients with infant botulism are constipated, and honey was a commonly recommended treatment for constipation. This finding was likely a noncausal association. Although honey has since been linked to infant botulism, and most parents are aware that honey should not be provided to babies, cases of infant botulism continue to occur.

A more compelling causal factor is an exposure to soil. Such contact, directly or through caregivers with occupational soil exposure (eg, caregivers employed in such fields as agriculture, landscaping, or road construction), exposes infants to botulism spores from the soil. Although some honey products might contain small amounts of botulism spores, soil is more ubiquitous and contains more botulism spores.

The pathogenesis is likely the ingestion of *C botulinum* spores, which then slowly proliferate and form small amounts of botulinum toxin, a known paralyzing toxin. Exposure initially results in bowel dysfunction and constipation, followed by poor feeding, weakness, hypotonia, and hyporeflexia. The botulinum toxin is a neuromuscular blocker. Aminoglycosides such as gentamicin are also weak neuromuscular blockers. Note that in this case, the patient was given gentamicin, which was promptly followed by respiratory arrest. The infant botulism caused weakness and impending respiratory failure, further aggravated by the gentamicin. Weak neonates are frequently admitted to rule out sepsis, and such patients are at risk for respiratory arrest if they actually have infant botulism and are given gentamicin.

Untreated, the botulinum toxin exposure continues and worsens. Long-term ventilation, nutrition, and life support permit the patient to eventually recover. Benefit may be conferred by antibiotic treatment and treatment with human botulinum immunoglobulin, but these benefits are variable. Infant botulism differs from adult botulism. In infant botulism, the infant ingests a few spores, which proliferate and slowly secrete small amounts of toxin, resulting in a slowly progressive paralysis. In adult botulism, an anaerobic environment, usually a defectively canned food, supports *C botulinum* proliferation and botulinum toxin production within the can. Once the can is opened and the food is consumed, a large amount of botulinum toxin is ingested, resulting in rapid onset of severe symptoms.

Recommended Reading

Gorelick MH, Blackwell CD. Neurologic emergencies. In: Fleisher GR, Ludwig S, Henretig FM, Ruddy RM, Silverman BK, eds. *Textbook of Pediatric Emergency Medicine.* 5th ed. Philadelphia, PA: Lippincott Williams & Wilkins; 2006:759–781

Ulrich DW. Infant botulism. In: Yamamoto LG, Inaba AS, Okamoto JK, Patronis ME, Yamashiroya VK, eds. *Case Based Pediatrics for Medical Students and Residents.* Honolulu, HI: University of Hawaii; 2004:550–551. Available at: http://www.hawaii.edu/medicine/pediatrics/pedtext. Accessed December 30, 2008

Chapter 41

Pallor, Listlessness, and Abnormal Respiratory Effort

Presentation

A previously healthy 3-month-old boy arrives by ambulance to the emergency department (ED) after an episode of listlessness and abnormal breathing. He had been well until an early morning feeding, after which he spit up and became listless with shallow respirations. His parents report that he appeared pale during the episode, and they indicate that he has had no preceding fever, respiratory or gastrointestinal symptoms, rash, injury, or seizures. The child's behavior, respiratory status, and color have now returned to normal. The paramedics describe normal vital signs and an uneventful transport.

On examination, the child is afebrile, vigorous, and well perfused, with strong pulses, normal vital signs, and normal room air oxyhemoglobin saturation (100%). Anterior fontanel is soft and flat, and his head circumference is 41 cm (50th percentile for age). Funduscopic examination is normal. He has clear, unlabored respirations and a soft, nontender abdomen. Skin examination reveals no bruising or other external signs of injury.

Discussion

Differential Diagnosis
- Near-miss sudden infant death syndrome
- Apparent life-threatening event
- Arrhythmia (long QT syndrome)
- Gastroesophageal reflux
- Drug ingestion
- Respiratory infection
- Sepsis
- Inflicted injury

Evaluation
At the very least, the events preceding this presentation constituted an apparent life-threatening event. Although the child is now asymptomatic, the unusual constellation of unexplained nonspecific symptoms (respiratory, gastrointestinal, and neurologic) are concerning for the possibility of a serious underlying medical or surgical disorder or occult injury. The events could not be easily explained by any common, benign event or discernible medical condition such as choking, breath holding, or bronchiolitis. Another worrisome possibility is head trauma, particularly inflicted.

Chest radiographs demonstrate no infiltrate, cardiomegaly, or fractures of the ribs or humeri. Screening laboratory tests include the following: white blood cells 14,500/μL, hemoglobin 11.2 g/dL, platelets 345,000/mcL, prothrombin time 11.0 seconds, partial thromboplastin time 26 seconds, and a normal chemistry panel. Computed tomography imaging reveals evidence of extraaxial blood in both frontal convexities, greater on the left than the right (figures 41-1, 41-2, and 41-3).

Treatment
The appearance of the fluid collections suggests subdural location. Although subdural effusions have been reported in rare medical conditions, inflicted head injury is the principal concern. The patient is admitted to the critical care unit for monitoring but requires no neurosurgical intervention, mechanical ventilation, or measures to decrease intracranial pressure.

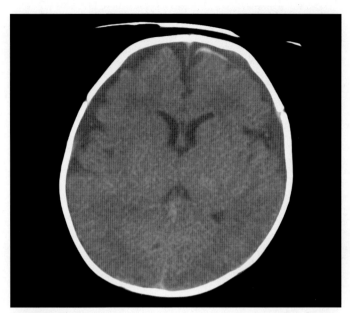

Figure 41-1

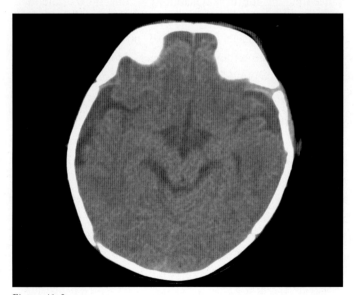

Figure 41-2

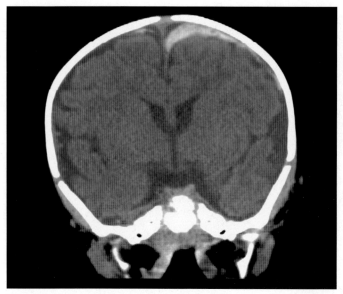

Figure 41-3

Magnetic resonance imaging confirms the abnormal collections of blood and reveals acute (on the order of days) and chronic (weeks to months) components. A radiographic skeletal survey reveals no fractures. An ophthalmology consultant finds no retinal hemorrhages. Urine organic acid screening reveals no evidence of underlying metabolic disorder.

A child protection evaluation concludes that the findings are the result of inflicted injury and the patient is discharged to foster care.

Keep in Mind

Although severe injury is unlikely to escape medical attention, inflicted head injury can manifest with subtle and nonspecific symptoms. About one third of children ultimately diagnosed with abusive head injury may have been examined by a physician one or more times previously for the same complaint. Independent risk factors for missed or delayed diagnosis of inflicted head injury include normal respiratory status, absence of seizures, absence of facial or scalp injury, and intact family status. Facial and scalp bruising is often attributed to accidents unrelated to the complaint.

Moreover, serious intracranial injury may be present in the complete absence of external bruising. Common alternative diagnoses before the discovery of inflicted injury include gastroenteritis, accidental injury, and miscellaneous medical conditions, including otitis media, seizure, gastroesophageal reflux, upper respiratory infection, and urinary tract infection.

Inflicted head injury should be considered in the differential diagnosis of infants who have symptoms of an apparent life-threatening event. Unexplained nonspecific symptoms in infants, even if resolved by the time of arrival to the ED, should prompt consideration of serious underlying conditions, including inflicted injury. Because serious intracranial injuries (subdural and subarachnoid hemorrhages or diffuse axonal injury) may result from a severe acceleration-deceleration mechanism which may occur with forceful shaking, the absence of external injury should not dissuade the clinician from pursuing the diagnosis of nonaccidental trauma.

Healthy nonambulatory children rarely incur bruises, lacerations, or fractures by accident. Intracranial injury, in particular, should not result from minor household accidents such as fall from a bed or other furniture and generally occurs as the consequence of a well-described and reliably witnessed major trauma mechanism.

Recommended Reading

Altman RL, Brand DA, Forman S, et al. Abusive head injury as a cause of apparent life-threatening events in infancy. *Arch Pediatr Adolesc Med.* 2003;157:1011–1015

Jenny C, Hymel KP, Ritzen A, Reinert SE, Hay TC. Analysis of missed cases of abusive head trauma. *JAMA.* 1999;281:621–626

Chapter 42

Ataxia With Rapidly Changing Mental Status

Presentation

A previously healthy 3-year-old girl is brought by ambulance to the emergency department (ED) because of new-onset ataxia and somnolence with dysarthria. She was asymptomatic and in completely good health until shortly before the family called 911. Within 15 to 30 minutes of her last clearly normal behavior, her family observed her to be increasingly clumsy. She rapidly became drowsy, and they feared that she might lose consciousness and stop breathing. A house guest has been visiting but the family thinks that all medications are inaccessible or in childproof containers. They have brought with them to the ED all of the medications they could locate. These include empty bottles of H1 and H2 histamine antagonists, a corticosteroid, and a benzodiazepine. Other bottles still contain antibiotics, acetaminophen, and other H1 and H2 histamine antagonists. All were found in their usual storage locations, and all appear securely closed. No additional agents are discovered after a rapid search of the house.

The patient is afebrile with normal vital signs and room air oxyhemoglobin saturation of 100%. Perfusion and ventilation are normal. She is alert and interactive for a brief period during initial examination. She reaches out for offered objects and attempts to speak in a dysarthric manner with both you and her mother. She has mild truncal and marked gait ataxia, but her strength is normal. There is no rash or nuchal rigidity.

Discussion

Differential Diagnosis

- Ingestion, either accidental or as the result of abuse or neglect
- Acute cerebellar ataxia
- Encephalitis
- Metabolic disturbance (eg, electrolyte disturbance, hypoglycemia)
- Hypoxia or hypercarbia
- Encephalopathy (eg, hepatic, renal)
- Central nervous system (CNS) mass lesion
- Trauma
- Intussusception

Evaluation

The differential diagnosis for new-onset ataxia is broad—and concerning if combined with altered mental status or respiratory function or perfusion. In this case, you think that ingestion appears to be the most likely scenario. However, given the nature of the medicines brought in by the parents or other medications that the visitor might have brought, the likelihood of significant intoxication by one of the reported medications appears low. Nonetheless, you proceed with a wide range of screening tests.

Laboratory tests of blood obtained during the start of an intravenous (IV) line reveal a normal complete blood cell count and differential, normal blood gas analysis, normal electrolytes and transaminases, and glucose 92 mg/dL. A urine toxicology test is negative for amphetamines and meth-amphetamines, phencyclidine, opiates, barbiturates, methadone, benzodi-azepines, cocaine, and cannabinoids. Acetaminophen and salicylate are undetectable. An electrocardiogram reveals no prolongation of QRS interval or any evidence of arrhythmia.

Treatment

The patient is kept fasting and maintenance IV fluids are begun. Initially, with no clinical evidence of trauma, CNS infection, or intraabdominal pathology, the patient is observed without further tests. Early during her ED stay, somnolence develops and persists, and her mother recalls the possibility of head injury during recent play. Computed tomography scan of the head is performed but is negative for intracranial pathology.

The continuing observation period is marked by episodes of uncharacteristic irritability alternating with somnolence. Lumbar puncture is considered, although your suspicion for meningitis or encephalitis is low. During discussion of the proposed procedure, the patient appears to resume normal behavior. Her gait improves significantly, with only mild remnant ataxia. Thereafter, she remains alert and interactive without further somnolence or irritability.

Despite the lack of clear cause for her symptoms, she is discharged to the care of her family with a plan for close observation. When they return home, the family learns that the houseguest had stored extended-release zolpidem tartrate (Ambien CR) in a suitcase and has since discovered that several tablets are missing.

Keep in Mind

Zolpidem, a nonbenzodiazepine hypnotic, preferentially binds to the type I benzodiazepine (GABA) receptor. Its rapid onset and short half-life make it useful for induction of sleep without the anxiolytic, anticonvulsant, or myorelaxant effects of benzodiazepines. The extended-release tablet provides rapid initial absorption with sustained plasma concentrations. Overdose results in CNS depression, and even at standard doses in adults, the most common adverse effects are dizziness and drowsiness. Respiratory depression is rare unless combined with other CNS depressants. Flumazenil may be useful in the treatment of respiratory depression resulting from zolpidem as long as an underlying seizure disorder or dangerous coingestion is not likely.

This case demonstrates the limitations of drug screening tests. Only a limited number of substances are included in any laboratory's panel. Zolpidem and many other sedative-hypnotics, including various classes of benzodiazepines, may escape detection by a routine drug screening test. When positive for a substance consistent with the clinical manifestation, laboratory drug screening tests may eliminate the need to investigate less likely causes and may lead to child protection measures if an illegal substance is detected. Rarely, the discovery of an unsuspected ingestion may lead to a specific antidote, such as N-acetylcysteine in the case of acetaminophen ingestion. However, for most ingestions, the management is supportive and based on a careful evaluation of the clinical presentation and other basic screening tests.

Toddlers and young children are at risk for preventable ingestion because of their exploratory behavior and interaction with their environment. Childproofing efforts may be subverted when a visitor brings medications into the home.

Recommended Reading

American Society of Health-System Pharmacists Inc. Zolpidem tartrate. In: McEvoy GK, ed. *AHFS Drug Information.* Bethesda, MD: American Society of Health-System Pharmacists Inc; 2003:2402–2405

Isaacman DJ, Trainor JL, Rothrock SG. Central nervous system. In: Gausche-Hill M, Fuchs S, Yamamoto L. *APLS: The Pediatric Emergency Medicine Resource.* 4th rev ed. Sudbury, MA: Jones and Bartlett Publishers; 2007:146–185

Lee DC. Sedative-hypnotics. In: Flomenbaum NE, Goldfrank LR, Hoffman RS, Howland MA, Lewin NA, Nelson LS, eds. *Goldfrank's Toxicologic Emergencies.* 8th ed. New York, NY: McGraw-Hill; 2006:1098–1111

Nelson DS. Coma and altered level of consciousness. In: Fleisher GR, Ludwig S, Henretig FM, Ruddy RM, Silverman BK. *Textbook of Pediatric Emergency Medicine.* 5th ed. Philadelphia, PA: Lippincott Williams & Wilkins; 2006:201–212

Chapter 43

Adolescent Unable to Be Aroused

Presentation

A 17-year-old boy is brought to the emergency department (ED) at night because he was not able to be aroused at home. He has been feeling ill since yesterday with lethargy and 5 episodes of vomiting. His mother checked him tonight and could not get him to respond. They carried him into the car and brought him to the ED. On arrival, he was walking with assistance. He was placed on the ED gurney and he made no further effort to move. There is no history of fever or seizures. He had also complained of mouth pain the previous day.

Past medical history indicates that he was previously healthy.

When you examine the patient, you record the following vital signs: axillary temperature 36.7°C, pulse 96 beats/min, respiration 14 breaths/min, blood pressure 100/60 mm Hg, and oxygen saturation 98% in room air. He is large and obese. He does not respond to verbal or painful stimuli. His oral mucosa is very dry with visible cracks on his tongue. His neck is supple. His heartbeat is regular; his heart is tachycardic with no murmurs. His lungs are clear and his abdomen is soft with bowel sounds. A neurologic examination is not easily performed because he is unresponsive and not moving his extremities. His color is good, but his extremities are cool. Capillary refill time is approximately 3 seconds.

Discussion

Differential Diagnosis

- Shock
- Coma
- Brain injury
- Brain hemorrhage
- Occult status epilepticus
- Encephalitis
- Diabetic ketoacidosis (DKA) coma
- Hypoglycemia
- Drug ingestion
- Sepsis
- Meningitis
- Hyperosmolar coma
- Alcohol intoxication

Evaluation

Laboratory evaluation is performed, with the following findings: bedside glucose greater than 400 mg/dL; arterial blood gas on O_2 by mask pH 7.00, P_{CO_2} 25 mm Hg, P_{O_2} 303 mm Hg, base excess -23, sodium 125 mmol/L, potassium 3.0 mmol/L, chloride 101 mmol/L, bicarbonate 4 mmol/L, serum ketones slightly increased, and glucose 1,800 mg/dL.

Complete blood count reveals white blood cells 16,000/μL, 3% bands, 60% segmented neutrophils, 37% lymphocytes, hemoglobin 15 g/dL, hematocrit 46%, and platelet count 450,000/μL.

Urinalysis is not performed because no urine was easily obtained.

The patient is diagnosed with new-onset diabetes mellitus with hyperosmolar coma and severe dehydration.

Treatment

Oxygen is administered by nonrebreather mask. Two intravenous lines are initiated and normal saline is infused rapidly in 20 mL/kg boluses. Treatment is initiated before the laboratory values are available. A trial dose of naloxone can be administered. Antibiotics can be administered for the possibility of sepsis, and acyclovir can be administered for the possibility of herpes encephalitis. Given the laboratory results shown previously, the patient is presenting with severe hyperglycemia and coma, most likely due to diabetes mellitus and nonketotic hyperosmolar coma. An insulin infusion is initiated.

New-onset diabetes mellitus often presents to the ED with classic symptoms of polyuria and polydipsia. However, most cases manifest as mild, moderate, or severe DKA. This patient has a glucose value that is much higher than what is usually seen with DKA and a low quantity of ketones. This manifestation is more consistent with diabetic hyperosmolar, nonketotic coma, known as a hyperglycemic hyperosmolar state (HHS). Patients with HHS typically have higher bicarbonate values than patients with DKA. Thus, this particular patient is not typical because of the extreme acidosis. However, severely ill HHS patients are likely to be extremely acidotic. This is a bad sign, and the risk of death is high. This patient was aggressively rehydrated, but shortly after he arrived at the ED, his hypotension worsened and he experienced refractory cardiac arrest.

Keep in Mind

Hyperglycemic hyperosmolar state patients tend to be patients with type 2 diabetes despite the extremely high glucose values. The reason for the absent or minimal ketosis is that a small amount of baseline pancreatic insulin production is often present. Lower amounts of insulin (approximately one tenth) can prevent lipolysis, but these low levels are inadequate to prevent hyperglycemia. This doesn't explain why some patients with type 1 diabetes develop HHS.

Although some patients with DKA can be managed on the hospital wards, patients with HHS are at higher risk of death and should be managed in an intensive care unit. The management of HHS patients is similar to the management of DKA patients in many ways; however, many therapeutic decisions are still controversial. Should insulin be given at a low dose or initially withheld? How rapidly should fluid be infused if the patient is severely dehydrated? Although there is some consensus in the management of DKA, there are fewer patients with HHS, and less information results in less consensus.

Recommended Reading

Agus MS. Endocrine emergencies. In: Fleisher GR, Ludwig S, Henretig FM,
    Ruddy RM, Silverman BK, eds. *Textbook of Pediatric Emergency
    Medicine.* 5th ed. Philadelphia, PA: Lippincott Williams & Wilkins;
    2006:1167–1192

Cochran JB, Walters S, Losek JD. Pediatric hyperglycemic hyperosmolar
    syndrome: diagnostic difficulties and high mortality rate. *Am J Emerg
    Med.* 2006;24:297–301

Glaser N, Enns GM, Kupperman N. Metabolic disease. In: Gausche-Hill M,
    Fuchs S, Yamamoto L, eds. *APLS: The Pediatric Emergency Medicine
    Resource.* 4th rev ed. Sudbury, MA: Jones and Bartlett Publishers;
    2007:186–207

Kitabchi AE, Nyenwe EA. Hyperglycemic crises in diabetes mellitus:
    diabetic ketoacidosis and hyperglycemic hyperosmolar state. *Endocrinol
    Metab Clin North Am.* 2006;35:725–751

Chapter 44

Severe Hypernatremia

Presentation

Paramedics respond to a 911 call and find a 3-year-old boy who is poorly responsive. He has poor respirations. His electrocardiogram shows a bradycardia with premature ventricular contractions. He is mask ventilated and his heart rate improves. Paramedics intubate him at the scene without sedative or paralytic agents. After the intubation he is noted to have fixed and dilated pupils, and his Glasgow coma score is 3. He is transported to the closest emergency department (ED).

According to the child's father, they were at the beach near the ocean 4 hours before calling the ambulance. The father states that the child was sitting in the water and began drinking salt water. The father told his son to stop, and he did. The family went home, where the child was playing and watching television. Three hours after this episode, while at home, he complained of some abdominal pain and vomited once. He then developed respiratory difficulty and rapidly worsened, prompting the 911 call.

Past medical history is not obtainable.

At arrival in the ED, examination of vital signs revealed the following: axillary temperature 36.4°C, pulse 120 beats/min, respiration 45 breaths/min (via bag ventilation through the endotracheal tube), blood pressure 80/60 mm Hg, and oxygen saturation 100%. He shows no significant neurologic response. His pupils are fixed and dilated. He is small for his age and emaciated in appearance.

Initial laboratory studies have the following results: arterial pH 7.02, Pco_2 51 mm Hg, Po_2 140 mm Hg, sodium 193 mmol/L, potassium 3.3 mmol/L, chloride 146 mmol/L, bicarbonate 12 mmol/L, glucose 300 mg/dL, blood urea nitrogen 28 mg/dL, and creatinine 0.7 mg/dL. A drug screen was negative. Complete blood count reveals white blood cells 14,200/µL,

61% segmented neutrophils, 11% bands, 26% lymphocytes, 3% monocytes, hemoglobin 10.8 g/dL, hematocrit 34.2%, and platelet count 330,000/μL.

He is provided intravenous (IV) fluids and furosemide. He is then transferred to a children's hospital for further management.

On arrival at the pediatric ED, his pupils are still fixed and dilated.

No neurologic response is noted. Retinal hemorrhages are noted on funduscopy.

His laboratory tests are repeated, with the following findings: sodium 179 mmol/L, potassium 3.3 mmol/L, chloride 148 mmol/L, bicarbonate 16 mmol/L, glucose 169 mg/dL, blood urea nitrogen 23 mg/dL, and creatinine 0.9 mg/dL.

Discussion

Differential Diagnosis
- Hypernatremia
- Coma
- Traumatic brain injury
- Salt poisoning
- Endocrinopathy (diabetes insipidus)
- Seizure with ischemic encephalopathy
- Failure to thrive (small for age)

Evaluation
A computed tomography (CT) scan of the brain is performed (Figure 44-1). The image on the left is taken through the orbits. This cut is significant for hemorrhages noted over the surface of the retina. The image on the right is taken through the brain and the lateral ventricles. Although IV contrast has not been administered, the falx appears to be prominent. This white enhancement represents hemorrhage in the interhemispheric space. It is most prominent posteriorly. This represents a posterior interhemispheric subdural hematoma. There is evidence of cerebral edema and a slight midline shift. This CT scan is pathognomonic of an abusive head injury. The retinal hemorrhages are also highly indicative of inflicted head injury.

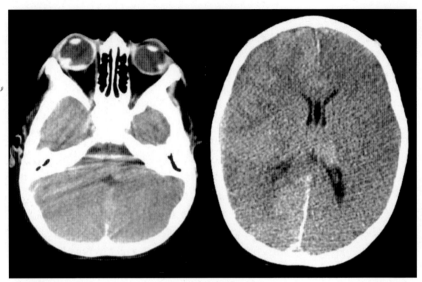

Figure 44-1

This degree of hypernatremia is not possible from drinking seawater for a short period. Saltwater near-drowning victims do not have this degree of hypernatremia. Whenever the history of events as described by the caregiver is not consistent with the clinical findings, child abuse should be suspected. In this case, the description of the child drinking some sea-water at the beach in the afternoon, playing happily later that afternoon, then being found in a near-arrest state a few minutes later by paramedics with extreme hypernatremia, retinal hemorrhages, and the posterior inter-hemispheric subdural hematoma noted at arrival at the hospital are an impossible sequence of events.

Retinal hemorrhages are usually identified on funduscopic examination. For medical and legal reasons, it may be best to have these substantiated by an ophthalmologist. In subtle cases, the retinal hemorrhages may not be seen on direct ophthalmoscopy; thus, an ophthalmologist is usually needed to perform indirect ophthalmoscopy. Most retinal hemorrhages are not visible on CT scan, so CT scan is not useful in ruling out the presence of retinal hemorrhages.

The finding of a prominent posterior falx on an unenhanced CT scan (no contrast) is indicative of a posterior interhemispheric subdural hematoma. In an infant, this is classically seen in shaken baby syndrome. Blood also enters the subarachnoid space. Thus, if a lumbar puncture is performed, it will most likely be grossly bloody.

Treatment

The hypernatremia in this case is extreme. Clinicians should be highly suspicious that this degree of hypernatremia may be of long standing. Thus, a rapid correction of this hypernatremia may be clinically detrimental; it may be best to correct this slowly. Clinical hydration and neurologic parameters should be followed closely to maintain a fluid balance most appropriate for the clinical situation. Rapid fluid and electrolyte shifts may result in cerebral edema. Fluid boluses may be required to correct hypovolemia, and diuretics may be necessary to manage cerebral edema. However, all such agents should be administered with extreme caution.

Keep in Mind

Deliberate poisoning of children by their caregivers is a recognized syndrome of child abuse. Sometimes, this is part of Munchausen syndrome by proxy, but in most instances, it is just another form of inflicted harm on a child. Nonaccidental salt poisoning is a common type of chronic poisoning administered to children by caregivers. Although many practitioners have not heard of this, it probably occurs more commonly than most believe. It may only come to medical attention if the poisoning results in severe hypernatremia.

Substantiated cases of salt poisoning are associated with severe hypernatremia, usually above 160 mEq/L. It is sometimes in excess of 200 mEq/L and is often in the range of 170 to 190 mEq/L. This finding is often found in association with other signs of physical abuse such as fractures, retinal hemorrhages, burns, failure to thrive, and emotional deprivation. In many of these instances, salt administration is used as a form of punishment.

For the serum sodium to be this high, the child must be deprived of water, salt must be forcibly administered, or both. Some mothers have been noted to put excessive amounts of salt in their infant's formula. Although 2 teaspoons of salt may not sound like much, this amount is capable of increasing a small infant's sodium level to 200 mmol/L, although the kidneys would generally excrete as much sodium as possible to prevent this from happening. Two teaspoons of salt have a strong taste, and when added to formula, infants will reject it. Thus, only when conventional fluids and formula are withheld would an infant be desperate enough to drink such salt-laden formula.

It is important to rule out organic causes of hypernatremia. Renal function should be ascertained, and normalization of the serum sodium under hospital or foster care with normal feedings should be documented. A urine sodium value obtained while the child is hypernatremic should be obtained. Hyperaldosteronism and diabetes insipidus are associated with inappropriately low urine sodium values, suggesting inappropriate sodium retention, while salt poisoning is associated with greatly increased urine sodium levels—the kidneys are attempting to correct the hypernatremia by excreting sodium. Hypernatremic dehydration resulting from gastroenteritis may mimic many of these findings; however, gastroenteritis and dehydration are usually associated with high blood urea nitrogen, whereas salt poisoning does not result in as much azotemia. Although hypernatremic dehydration generally results in only modest sodium increases, salt poisoning is associated with extremely high sodium measurements.

The absence of polyuria by history makes diabetes insipidus less likely. However, the presence of polydipsia is often seen in salt poisoning in an attempt to compensate for the hypernatremia or fluid deprivation. Such children have been observed to lick water off windows and to drink from puddles, toilets, and fish tanks.

Although accidentally (or out of ignorance) administering undiluted formula concentrate to infants usually results in hypernatremia, this type of unintentional hypernatremia is usually not as extreme, and the other associated findings, such as failure to thrive or inflicted injuries, are not present.

Although initial interviews with parents guilty of poisoning their children with salt did not reveal a willful attempt to harm the child, in repeated interviews months later, some parents confessed to wanting to kill their child. In a few instances when salt-poisoned children were returned to their parents, the salt-poisoning behavior recurred despite the parents' knowledge that this was harmful. This suggests that such perpetrators are severely disturbed, and these children should be placed in protected environments away from the perpetrator.

Although speculative, it is likely that there are lesser degrees of salt poisoning that result in only modest or transient hypernatremia, or hypernatremia that is difficult to distinguish from hypernatremic dehydration caused by gastroenteritis. This may not be very harmful unless it leads to more severe salt poisoning. It is probably prudent to routinely question the caregivers of any child with even mild hypernatremia for the possibility of salt administration. If this response to inquiry is suspicious, or the child has any other high-risk factors (eg, failure to thrive, fractures, burns, inappropriate social behavior, developmental delays), frequent clinical and laboratory follow-up monitoring for signs of salt poisoning or other forms of child abuse and neglect would be in the child's best interest. Reporting a case to the local child protective authorities would enable one to determine whether any other suspicious events have ever been reported about the child.

In the case of this patient, one could speculate that this child was chronically salt poisoned. He also endured an acute shaking episode resulting in cerebral and retinal hemorrhaging; such shaking may even be chronic. This type of injury results in axonal shearing and cerebral edema. If this was acute and severe enough, it likely accounts for his vomiting and rapid decline. Rapid changes in serum osmolarity may have also contributed to the cerebral edema. The father's history of events could not possibly account for the child's clinical findings. This child was small for his age, and he demonstrated clear failure to thrive, weighing a mere 10 kg at age 3 years. Despite his small stature, he was not brought in for routine medical care. This family was previously known to the local child protective services, who had received reports of suspected child abuse and neglect in the past.

Recommended Reading

Bays J. Child abuse by poisoning. In: Reece RM. *Child Abuse: Medical Diagnosis and Management.* Philadelphia, PA: Lea & Febinger; 1994:87–88

Dyer C. Mother found guilty in case of fabricated illness. *BMJ.* 2005;330:497

Meadow R. Non-accidental salt poisoning. *Arch Dis Child.* 1993;68: 448–452

Southall DP, Plunkett MC, Banks MW, Falkov AF, Samuels MP. Covert video recordings of life-threatening child abuse: lessons for child protection. *Pediatrics.* 1997;100:735–760

Yamamoto LG. Severe hypernatremia—salt poisoning. In: Yamamoto LG, Inaba AS, DiMauro R, eds. *Radiology Cases in Pediatric Emergency Medicine.* Vol 3, case 14. August 1995. Available at: http://www.hawaii.edu/medicine/pediatrics/pemxray/v3c14.html. Accessed December 30, 2008

Chapter 45

Chickenpox and Agitation

Presentation

A 2-year-old girl is brought to the emergency department (ED) by her mother because of fever, fussiness, agitation, and chickenpox. The onset of the chickenpox was 2 days ago. She has had fever for 2 days with a maximum temperature of 39.5°C yesterday. She has many itchy lesions and has vomited twice today. She has been treated with ibuprofen with good fever control. She has also been treated with diphenhydramine and calamine lotion.

Past medical history is unremarkable, except that this family has refused most immunizations.

Your examination reveals the following vital signs: rectal temperature 38.6°C, pulse 185 beats/min, respiration 28 breaths/min while crying, blood pressure unobtainable, and oxygen saturation 99% in room air.

She is agitated and fussy, but not obviously toxic. She has an appearance of slight redness (erythroderma). Her eyes are tearing with mild conjunctival injection. Her pupils are difficult to see because of her agitation, but they appear to be large. Her oral mucosa is moist. Her tympanic membranes are slightly red. It is difficult to check for neck rigidity because she is so agitated. Heart is tachycardic with no obvious murmur. Lungs are clear. Abdomen is soft and flat with normal bowel sounds. Her liver edge is difficult to identify. She has no inguinal hernias. External genitalia are normal. Color and perfusion are good. Capillary refill is 1.5 to 2 seconds. Muscle tone and strength are good. She has many varicella lesions in different stages of healing (vesicles and early crusts). Some of the lesions appear impetiginous, with a golden, slightly purulent discharge. Residual calamine lotion is present on her skin. Although there is a slight redness to her skin, it does not appear to be like sandpaper, but this might be difficult to appreciate because of all the varicella lesions. Her skin feels warm and is without diaphoresis.

Discussion

Differential Diagnosis

- Varicella
- Impetigo with group A streptococci or *Staphylococcus aureus*
- Erythroderma due to scarlet fever, toxic shock, or anticholinergic overdose
- Agitation due to Reye syndrome, encephalitis, or anticholinergic overdose
- Tachycardia due to agitation, fever, anticholinergic overdose, or shock

Evaluation

An intravenous (IV) line is started, and the patient is given IV ceftriaxone, clindamycin, and acyclovir. She is observed in the ED for a period of 4 hours. The purpose of this prolonged observation period is to determine whether her clinical condition improves or worsens. If Reye syndrome or toxic shock is present, her condition is likely to worsen during the observation period. If benign scarlet fever is the cause of her erythroderma, her clinical condition is likely to remain stable. If her symptoms are due to an anticholinergic overdose, her clinical condition is likely to improve as the effect of excessive diphenhydramine wears off.

A chest radiograph shows clear lungs and a normal cardiac silhouette. An electrocardiogram shows a sinus tachycardia with a heart rate of 180 beats/min and excessive muscle artifact because of movement and agitation. Complete blood count shows a white blood cell count of 12,500/μL with 65% segmented neutrophils, 11% bands, 20% lymphocytes, 4% monocytes, hemoglobin 13.1 g/dL, and platelet count 360,000/μL. Laboratory values are as follows: ammonia 35 μg/dL (normal), glucose 110 mg/dL, sodium 136 mmol/L, potassium 4.1 mmol/L, chloride 100 mmol/L, and bicarbonate 20 mmol/L. C-reactive protein and erythrocyte sedimentation rate values are low.

Her erythroderma resolves as her temperature declines. Her agitation also resolves and she now appears to be alert, active, cooperative, and playful.

On further questioning, you discover that the calamine lotion that her mother has been applying is actually a combination product that contains calamine plus topical diphenhydramine (Caladryl). Because she has been taking diphenhydramine by mouth plus topical diphenhydramine applied over many open skin lesions, you conclude that she is at high risk of absorbing an overdose of diphenhydramine.

She is diagnosed with varicella, a diphenhydramine overdose, and secondary infections with *S aureus* and group A streptococcus.

Treatment
She is discharged from the ED and prescribed clindamycin, acyclovir, and antipyretics.

Keep in Mind
Although varicella is fairly uncommon as a result of high immunization rates, susceptible children can easily be exposed to someone with zoster. Many parents believe that herd immunity will protect their children. For pertussis and varicella, however, children are still exposed to substantial disease reservoirs.

Treating varicella with acyclovir has been shown to be of little benefit if it is started late, as in this case. Some children will develop complex or extensive varicella, and it is unclear whether initiating acyclovir therapy even after 48 hours will benefit such children. Acyclovir is relatively benign and not too expensive. Thus, weighing the potential small benefit against minimal risk potentially justifies its use in this case.

Some parents believe that washing the varicella lesions helps to spread them around more; thus, it is common for children of such parents to not be bathed properly during a course of varicella. This results in poor skin cleansing and secondary infections with group A streptococci and *S aureus*. These 2 organisms can cause scarlet fever, toxic shock syndrome, or both, and result in a modest erythroderma. Scarlet fever is relatively benign, but toxic shock can be fatal. These 2 conditions can be difficult to distinguish on initial examination; however, an observation period of several hours will often yield different clinical outcomes that can help the clinician distinguish between the two. Rapid improvement and continued stability suggest scarlet fever, while persistent vital sign abnormalities, sensation of weakness, and other evidence of perfusion compromise increase the likelihood of early toxic shock syndrome, necessitating the need for intensive care hospitalization and potentially the initiation of inotropic agents.

Reye syndrome is seen much less commonly. Its association with aspirin use has resulted in a dramatic decline in aspirin use in children, which has resulted in a dramatic decline in Reye syndrome. It is characterized by fatty changes in the liver as well as encephalopathy that often leads to coma. Common signs and symptoms include vomiting, agitation, and irrational behavior, with progression to lethargy, seizures, and coma. Reye syndrome classically occurs in a series of stages progressing from agitation and restlessness to lethargy, confusion, seizures, decorticate rigidity, decerebrate rigidity, coma, areflexia, dilated pupils, and respiratory arrest, with an isoelectric electroencephalogram. Early laboratory findings include hyperammonemia, high liver enzymes, and hypoglycemia.

Diphenhydramine overdose results in an anticholinergic overdose toxidrome commonly remembered by the following device: red as a beet, blind as a bat, mad as a hatter, dry as a bone, and hot as a hare. Other findings may include tachycardia, hypertension, tachypnea, hallucinations, seizures, hypoactive bowel sounds, dry mouth, and urinary retention. This patient is most likely to have had an overdose of diphenhydramine resulting in an anticholinergic toxidrome with erythroderma (red as a beet), pupillary dilation (blind as a bat), severe agitation and irritability (mad as a hatter), absent perspiration (anhydrosis, dry as a bone), and fever (hot as a hare). This resulted from a full dose of oral diphenhydramine in conjunction with topical diphenhydramine applied over multiple open lesions, resulting in an overdose. The standard pediatric dose of diphenhydramine is 5 mg/kg per day divided into 4 doses provided every 6 hours, which is 1.25 mg/kg per dose. For an 80-kg adult, the dose would be 100 mg. Most adults will take a 25-mg dose, or 50 mg at the most. Thus pediatric dosing of diphenhydramine is already high. When coupled with topical diphenhydramine, this can easily result in an overdose.

Recommended Reading

Boldt DW. Reye syndrome. In: Yamamoto LG, Inaba AS, Okamoto JK, Patronis ME, Yamashiroya VK, eds. *Case Based Pediatrics for Medical Students and Residents.* Honolulu, HI: University of Hawaii; 2004:580–582. Available at: http://www.hawaii.edu/medicine/pediatrics/pedtext. Accessed December 30, 2008

Erickson TB. Toxicology: ingestions and smoke inhalation. In: Gausche-Hill M, Fuchs S, Yamamoto L, eds. *APLS: The Pediatric Emergency Medicine Resource.* 4th rev ed. Sudbury, MA: Jones and Bartlett Publishers; 2007:234–267

Inaba AS. Toxicology. In: Yamamoto LG, Inaba AS, Okamoto JK, Patronis ME, Yamashiroya VK, eds. *Case Based Pediatrics for Medical Students and Residents.* Honolulu, HI: University of Hawaii; 2004:478–483. Available at: http://www.hawaii.edu/medicine/pediatrics/pedtext. Accessed December 30, 2008

Osterhoudt KC, Ewald MB, Shannon M, Henretig FM. Toxicologic emergencies. In: Fleisher GR, Ludwig S, Henretig FM, Ruddy RM, Silverman BK, eds. *Textbook of Pediatric Emergency Medicine.* 5th ed. Philadelphia, PA: Lippincott Williams & Wilkins; 2006:951–1007

Vincent JM. Staphylococcal and streptococcal toxic shock syndromes. In: Yamamoto LG, Inaba AS, Okamoto JK, Patronis ME, Yamashiroya VK, eds. *Case Based Pediatrics for Medical Students and Residents.* Honolulu, HI: University of Hawaii; 2004:199–203. Available at: http://www.hawaii.edu/medicine/pediatrics/pedtext. Accessed December 30, 2008

Chapter 46

Oncology Patient With Abdominal Pain and Swelling

Presentation

An 8-year-old boy is brought to the emergency department (ED) for right-sided abdominal swelling of 2 weeks' duration. The mass is painless and fluctuates in size, decreasing in the supine position. The patient denies any fevers, chills, vomiting, or diarrhea. The patient also denies abdominal pain, respiratory complaints, urinary tract symptoms, and other medical problems.

Four months previously, he was found to have a cerebellar medulloblastoma, after presenting with a 2-week history of headache, head tilt, and difficulty walking. He underwent partial resection and subsequently required placement of a ventriculoperitoneal shunt to relieve worsening hydrocephalus. His current therapy includes cranial radiation, dexamethasone, and an outpatient chemotherapy regimen. Adjunctive therapy includes trimethoprim sulfamethoxazole and ranitidine.

He has normal vital signs and is alert, afebrile, and well perfused, resting comfortably in bed. His scalp has a palpable shunt with no signs of infection and no fluid collection. His pupils are equal and reactive to light with normal extraocular movements. The abdomen is soft, nontender, and nondistended, with no organomegaly. On the right midabdomen, a surgical incision appears to be healing well without surrounding erythema or edema. A large mass approximately 10 × 10 cm arises in the vicinity of the wound and is easily compressible and nontender. Neurologic examination is normal.

Discussion

Differential Diagnosis

- Postoperative complications (eg, hernia, partial wound dehiscence)
- Postoperative infection
- Opportunistic infection
- Metastatic disease

Evaluation

The results of the laboratory evaluation (leukocyte count 9,600/μL, erythrocyte sedimentation rate 14 mm/hr, and C-reactive protein <0.3 mg/dL) reduce the likelihood that the swelling is caused by infection or inflammatory complications. A cranial computed tomography (CT) scan reveals no evidence of shunt malfunction, and the plain film shunt series reveals no

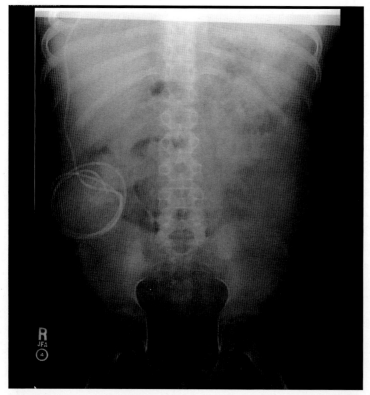

Figure 46-1

disruption or displacement of the cranial portion. The distal portion of the tubing overlies the abdomen but appears tightly coiled (Figure 46-1). Abdominal CT demonstrates the caudal tip of the shunt to be external to the peritoneal cavity, with fluid collection external to the abdominal muscle layers (Figure 46-2).

Treatment
The patient undergoes operative revision of the distal portion of the shunt. The distal portion is found coiled within a large extraperitoneal pseudocyst and is placed into the peritoneal cavity without complication. Cultures from the pseudocyst cavity are negative for bacterial growth.

Keep in Mind
Migration of a ventricular drainage catheter is a rare but important complication that may manifest as a mass effect or malfunction. Extraabdominal cerebrospinal fluid pseudocysts with or without neurologic symptoms have resulted from migration of catheter tips into the labium majus through the

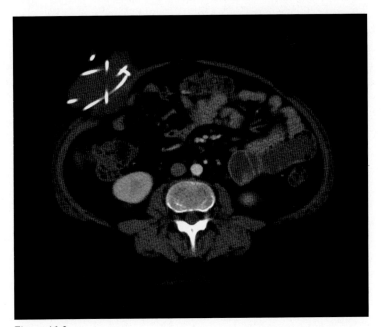

Figure 46-2

canal of Nuck, into the subgaleal space, out of the peritoneal insertion site, and into the breast surrounding a previously placed implant. Rarely, the shunt tip may perforate a hollow viscus with attendant risk of shunt infection or intraabdominal infection.

Recommended Reading

Akcora B, Serarslan Y, Sangun O. Bowel perforation and transanal protrusion of a ventriculoperitoneal shunt catheter. *Pediatr Neurosurg.* 2006;42:129–131

Gan PY, Singhal A. Complete upward migration of the peritoneal end of a ventriculoperitoneal shunt into the subgaleal space. *Pediatr Neurosurg.* 2006;42:404–405

Gan YC, Steinbok P. Migration of the peritoneal tip of a ventriculoperitoneal catheter causing shunt malfunction. Case illustration. *J Neurosurg.* 2006;105(2 suppl):153

Spector JA, Culliford AT, Post NH, Weiner H, Levine JP. An unusual case of cerebrospinal fluid pseudocyst in a previously augmented breast. *Ann Plast Surg.* 2005;54:85–87

Yuksel KZ, Senoglu M, Yuksel M, Ozkan KU. Hydrocele of the canal of Nuck as a result of a rare ventriculoperitoneal shunt complication. *Pediatr Neurosurg.* 2006;42:193–196

Chapter 47

Agitation Following Minor Head Trauma

Presentation

While playing during recess at school, a 5-year-old girl collided with her friend and fell backward, striking the back of her head on the grass. This was witnessed by her teacher, who took her to see the school nurse. She seemed to be normal, and after a brief rest in the nurse's room, she was returned to class. Thirty minutes later, she vomited once in class and was sent back to the nurse, who called her mother at work to pick her daughter up early from school. There were no complaints of headache or further nausea. Her mother picked her up and was driving home when the child's behavior gradually became combative and agitated. Instead of driving to her doctor's office, she drove to the emergency department to have her child evaluated.

Past medical history is not contributory.

Your examination reveals the following vital signs: temperature 37°C, pulse 150 beats/min, respiration 30 breaths/min, blood pressure unobtainable, and oxygen saturation 100% in room air. She is very agitated and combative. She does not respond to verbal commands from her mother or the staff. She does not appear to recognize or focus on her mother. Her head shows no evidence of external head trauma. Her ears are normal. Her pupils are difficult to fully assess, but they are large. Her neck is difficult to assess. Her heart is tachycardic without murmurs. Her lungs are clear. Her abdomen has normal bowel sounds. She moves all her extremities well.

Discussion

Differential Diagnosis
- Head injury
- Concussion
- Transient cortical blindness
- Drug ingestion

Evaluation
No immediate treatment is provided, although intravenous access may be considered. No laboratory work is truly necessary here unless drug ingestion or exposure is suspected.

A computed tomography (CT) scan of her head is performed and reveals no abnormalities. By this time, she has calmed down and is no longer agitated and combative. Optokinetic nystagmus testing is negative.

Treatment
A diagnosis of transient cortical blindness is made, and she is hospitalized for observation. Approximately 5 hours after her CT scan, her behavior normalizes. She begins speaking to her parents, and she interacts normally with the environment.

Keep in Mind
Transient cortical blindness is an unusual phenomenon that follows relatively minor head trauma. Initially, the patient experiences minor head trauma and seems to be fine. There might be some mild concussion symptoms. A proposed mechanism is that autoregulation of cerebral blood flow to the occipital cortex is disturbed by this trauma. In a phenomenon similar to migraine headaches, occipital cerebral blood flow is temporarily diminished, and temporary blindness follows. Agitated behavior, an inability to visually focus, and poor recognition of the environment are typical findings. A CT scan of the brain is important to rule out the possibility of more severe traumatic brain injury. Once a normal CT scan and a benign history of head trauma are confirmed, a benign outcome is likely. Optokinetic nystagmus is horizontal nystagmus that can be elicited by

passing a vertically striped sheet (Figure 47-1) horizontally in front of the patient's eyes at reading distance. Horizontal nystagmus is a normal finding when this is done. The absence of horizontal nystagmus when this optokinetic sheet is passed in front of the eyes indicates the lack of the visual stimulus entering or processing in the brain. This test can be used to determine whether the patient can see.

The terms *cortical blindness* and *cerebral blindness* are used when blindness is evident without eye pathology. Acutely, these terms are generally used when the pupillary response is normal. In some cases of transient cortical blindness caused by minor head trauma, the pupils can appear to be fixed and dilated. This is inconsistent with transtentorial herniation because these patients are generally awake and agitated. The cause of this pupillary dilation in some patients has been postulated to be a sympathetic discharge from the ciliospinal reflex. The pupils are actually large and difficult to constrict, rather than truly fixed and dilated.

There are many causes of cortical blindness. Many of these are vascular disturbances. Most are not benign. In the cases that have been reviewed in the literature, a benign outcome is predicted when the head trauma is minor and brain imaging studies are normal.

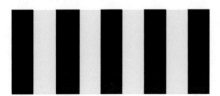

Figure 47-1

Recommended Reading

Gjerris F, Mellemgaard L. Transient cerebral blindness in head injury. *Acta Neurol Scand.* 1969;45:623–631

Rodriguez A, Lozano JA, del Pozo D, Homar Paez J. Post-traumatic transient cortical blindness. *Int Ophthalmol.* 1993;17:277–283

Yamamoto LG, Bart RD. Transient blindness following mild head trauma. Criteria for a benign outcome. *Clin Pediatr (Phila).* 1988;27:479–483

Chapter 48

Skull Fracture, Lethargy, and Vomiting

Presentation

A 7-month-old girl is brought to the emergency department with a chief complaint of a growing lump on the side of her head. She fell off the couch 6 days ago when a cousin was babysitting. There was no loss of consciousness or drowsiness noted and the child's behavior was unchanged, so no medical attention was sought. Two days later (4 days ago), her mother noted a lump developing on the right side of the infant's head. Today, she feels that the lump is very soft, and to her it feels like "the brain is sticking out." There is no history of vomiting or other trauma.

Past medical history is negative.

Examination reveals the following vital signs: rectal temperature 37.5°C, pulse 140 beats/min, respiration 36 breaths/min, and blood pressure 75/40 mm Hg. The infant is alert and active, and she is in no distress. Her anterior fontanelle is flat. A 10-cm region of soft swelling is noted over the right parietal region. Pupils are equal and reactive, and red reflex is present bilaterally. Her fundi are difficult to view. Examination of tympanic membranes reveals no blood. The patient's nose is clear, and the mouth is clear and moist. The neck is nontender and supple. The patient's heartbeat is regular without murmurs. Lungs are clear. The trunk does not show evidence of bruising. The patient's abdomen is soft and flat with active bowel sounds. No abdominal tenderness or masses are present. No hernias are present, and genitalia are normal. The patient's extremities lack swelling, deformity, or bruising and the patient uses them well. The infant's tone is good.

Discussion

Differential Diagnosis
- Subgaleal hematoma
- Underlying skull fracture
- Accidental trauma
- Child abuse
- Brain injury

Evaluation
A skull series is obtained (Figure 48-1). Clinically, this infant appears to have a subgaleal hematoma. These usually are brought to medical attention several days after the patient experiences an underlying skull fracture. The manifestation is often not immediate because the hemorrhage from the fracture forms a tight and palpably rigid swelling under the aponeurosis of Galen layer of the scalp. As blood from the hematoma is resorbed, the swelling softens. This soft spot on the infant's head is then noted by parents, often prompting a visit to a physician. In most instances, there are no complications because several days have elapsed since the head trauma incident without the infant exhibiting any signs or symptoms of brain injury. Radiographs of the skull would most often not alter your

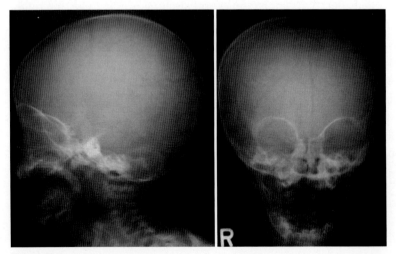

Figure 48-1

clinical approach except in a case such as this. In older children, a small
linear fracture under a subgaleal hematoma, found several days after the
head trauma event, is usually not serious. However, this patient is very
young, and the fracture visible on this radiograph is extensive.

This skull series shows extensive fractures of the right parietal skull.
One would expect to see a simple linear fracture in this region if the
trauma were accidental or benign. Additionally, there are extensive
fractures over the occipital skull and the contralateral parietal skull as
well. A simple fall off a couch could not possibly account for all these
fractures. Child abuse is overwhelmingly likely. A computed tomography (CT) scan of the brain is performed.

A high CT scan cut shows a bone window on the left and a brain window
on the right (Figure 48-2). The open anterior fontanelle is noted at the top
of both images. The large right parietal scalp swelling (subgaleal hematoma)
is noted. The bone window on the left shows a large right parietal fracture.
A smaller left parietal fracture is also evident. The coronal sutures are visible. There are several lucencies in the occiput. Two of these are the lamb-
doidal sutures, and the others are occipital fractures. The brain is normal.
Lower cuts do not demonstrate cerebral hemorrhages or edema. A posterior

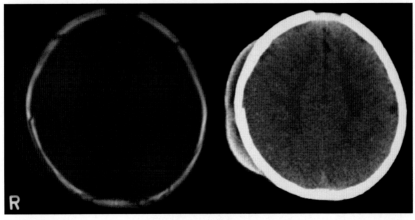

Figure 48-2

interhemispheric subdural hematoma is not evident on the lower cuts. This finding would be indicative of shaken baby syndrome.

A skeletal survey is obtained. No other fractures are identified on this skeletal survey. Only limited views are shown in Figure 48-3.

Because of the likelihood of child abuse and the potential for repeated abusive head trauma, the infant is hospitalized and child protective services are notified. During hospitalization, this infant does well. There is good weight gain, and her neurologic function and developmental evaluation are normal. A retina examination performed by an ophthalmologist is negative for hemorrhages.

On hospital day 3, she is noted to be less active than she has been, and she vomits 3 times. Abdominal examination is negative. She vomits again and is noted to be lethargic. A nasogastric tube is placed. A repeat CT scan of the brain is obtained to rule out a hemorrhage. The repeat CT scan fails to find any brain abnormalities. The skull fractures and scalp swelling are unchanged.

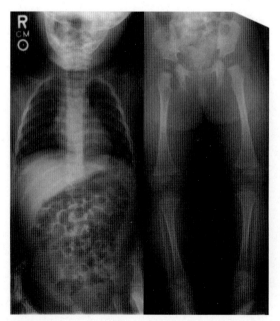

Figure 48-3

An abdominal series is ordered as part of her evaluation (Figure 48-4). The supine view is on the left and the upright view is on the right. This abdominal series shows a paucity of bowel gas. A nasogastric tube is placed in the stomach. The paucity of gas is quite remarkable and associated with several air-fluid levels, highly suspicious of a bowel obstruction. Such a paucity of gas associated with a bowel obstruction in a young child is highly suggestive of intussusception. The right upper quadrant shows a hint of a mass or target sign. The liver edge is obscured, which is known as absence of the subhepatic angle. The presence of these signs is highly suggestive of intussusception.

This infant actually developed an intussusception during a hospitalization for abusive head trauma. On the skeletal survey taken at admission, her abdominal radiograph shows a normal bowel gas pattern. She evidently developed intussusception while in the hospital, likely unrelated to the initial abuse events.

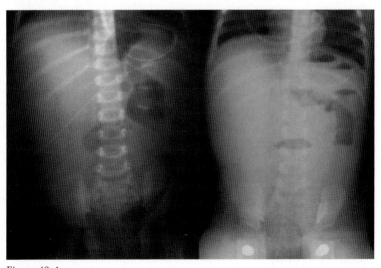

Figure 48-4

Treatment

A contrast enema confirmed the intussusception. It could not be reduced with hydrostatic pressure. She underwent a surgical reduction of the intussusception. There were no surgical findings to suggest that the intussusception was related to child abuse in any way. She recovered well and was discharged to foster care.

Keep in Mind

The terms *cephalohematoma* and *subgaleal hematoma* are often used interchangeably, but technically, a cephalohematoma is subperiosteal, whereas a subgaleal hematoma is beneath the aponeurosis of Galen. Cephalohematomas generally do not cross suture lines and they most often occur in newborns during a vaginal delivery. Subgaleal hematomas often occur in conjunction with a skull fracture.

The diagnosis of intussusception is an important diagnosis in pediatric emergency medicine. Because it occurs almost exclusively in young children, establishing the diagnosis is difficult, although intussusception diagnosed early has a better outcome than one diagnosed late. The clinical presentation falls into 1 of 2 major categories. The more common presentation is vomiting with severe intermittent (colicky) abdominal pain. The child appears to have severe cramps as manifested by discomfort and irritability. The painful episode subsides and then recurs every 10 to 40 minutes. The less common presentation is lethargy. This presentation is more often seen in infants with intussusception, rather than in children older than 12 months.

The radiographic findings of intussusception include several classic signs known as the target sign, the crescent sign, absence of the subhepatic angle, and a paucity of gas bowel obstruction. Because the most common type of intussusception occurs in the ileocecal region, the right side of the abdomen is often the area of focus. Small bowel intussusceptions (eg, ileoileal) are more difficult to diagnose. Although positive plain film radiographs are highly predictive of intussusception, negative plain film radiographs cannot usually be relied on to rule out the presence of intussusception. An abdominal ultrasound or a contrast enema has greater diagnostic accuracy.

The radiograph in Figure 48-5 demonstrates the target and crescent signs. The target sign resembles a faint doughnut shape in the right upper quadrant. The target sign is almost always in the right upper quadrant. It obscures the liver edge, resulting in absence of the subhepatic angle. The target sign is subtle and not easily recognized unless one is specifically searching for it.

The crescent sign is caused by the intussusceptum (leading point of the intussusception) protruding into a gas-filled pocket. In this case, the location of the crescent sign suggests that the intussusception has intussuscepted up the ascending colon and across most of the transverse colon.

The radiograph in Figure 48-6 shows another patient with intussusception. There is a target sign in the right upper quadrant. The target sign is subtle, but it again resembles a doughnut in the right upper quadrant. This radiographic appearance is due to alternating layers of fat and bowel tissue. The left upper quadrant demonstrates a crescent sign. In this case, the crescent sign more closely resembles the shape of a classic crescent, unlike in Figure 48-5.

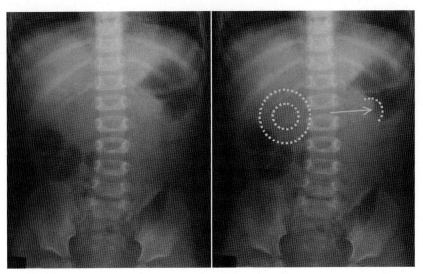

Figure 48-5

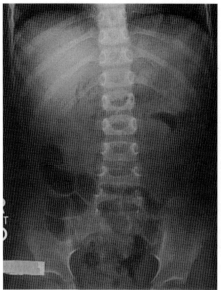

In the radiograph in Figure 48-7, the intussusceptum is pointing upward at the hepatic flexure. Most of the transverse colon is gas filled, permitting the visualization of the intussusceptum. In this case, the crescent sign is clearly not crescent shaped; rather, it manifests as the intussusceptum protruding into a gas-filled pocket. The crescent sign does not have to be crescent shaped.

Figure 48-6

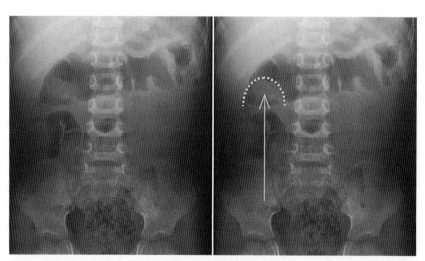

Figure 48-7

Recommended Reading

Yamamoto LG. Lethargy and vomiting following child abuse. In: Yamamoto LG, Inaba AS, DiMauro R, eds. *Radiology Cases in Pediatric Emergency Medicine.* Vol 5, case 10. October 1996. Available at: http://www.hawaii.edu/medicine/pediatrics/pemxray/v5c10.html. Accessed December 30, 2008

Young LL, Yamamoto LG. The stomach flu?—the target, crescent, and absent liver edge signs. In: Yamamoto LG, Inaba AS, DiMauro R, eds. *Radiology Cases in Pediatric Emergency Medicine.* Vol 1, case 2. November 1994. Available at: http://www.hawaii.edu/medicine/pediatrics/pemxray/v1c02.html. Accessed December 30, 2008

Chapter 49

Headache, Eye Pain, and Decreased Responsiveness

Presentation

A previously healthy 16-year-old boy reports left eye pain that began 10 days ago in a vaguely described periorbital location. Now he is experiencing greater pain intensity in a more well-localized distribution above the orbit and in the frontal region. He has experienced no head or ocular trauma. At the beginning of the illness, he underwent an evaluation at another hospital and received a prescription for a serotonin-receptor agonist for presumed migraine headaches. Subsequently, he developed intermittent low-grade fevers that are neither documented nor well described. He appears lethargic to other family members and has vomited today and several times earlier in the illness. Neither the patient nor any relatives have a prior history of migraines or other headache syndromes.

He is alert and well perfused with a temperature of 38.3°C and otherwise normal vital signs. He is cooperative but appears somewhat aloof and slow to respond to questions and commands. His neurologic examination is otherwise normal. Funduscopic examination reveals no papilledema. Slit lamp examination reveals a small, round lesion on his left cornea that does not stain with fluorescein. His anterior chamber is otherwise normal. He has no rash or nuchal rigidity.

Discussion

Differential Diagnosis

- Migraine
- Orbital disease (eg, foreign body, occult trauma, abscess, glaucoma)
- Sinusitis
- Central nervous system infection (eg, meningitis, parameningeal infection)
- Metabolic disturbance, especially hypoglycemia
- Hypoxia
- Seizures
- Drug ingestion

Evaluation

Previous treating clinicians have suggested that the headaches result from migraine and possible vision problems, and your patient's detachment may be typical of his usual behavior. However, because this patient's symptoms are persistent and remain unexplained, computed tomography (CT) imaging of the head and blood chemistry studies are requested. A complete blood count and toxicology screening are ordered. Visual acuity is normal. Results of laboratory studies include white blood cell count of 15,800/μL (78% neutrophils, 9% lymphocytes, and 13% monocytes), hemoglobin 14.7 g/dL, platelets 376,000/μL, normal electrolytes with no acidosis, glucose 112 mg/dL, normal transaminases, and a negative urine drug screen. Computed tomography images reveal a contrast-enhancing, convex left frontal lesion with an air-fluid level consistent with an epidural abscess (Figure 49-1). Associated findings include left frontal and ethmoid sinusitis (figures 49-2 and 49-3).

Treatment

The patient receives ceftriaxone and vancomycin in the emergency department before admission to the pediatric intensive care unit, where he continues to receive vancomycin and meropenem in addition to dexamethasone. In a combined procedure by the otolaryngology and neurosurgery services, the patient undergoes a left frontal craniotomy, abscess evacuation, and left frontal sinus trephination.

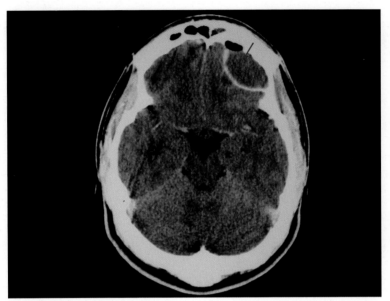

Figure 49-1

After surgery, the patient recovers rapidly and demonstrates no systemic signs of infection or neurologic abnormalities. Samples taken from the abscess and sinus are cultured and grow *Streptococcus pneumoniae* sensitive to penicillin and ceftriaxone. The patient receives a percutaneous central catheter to complete a 6-week outpatient course of ceftriaxone. He finishes a tapering course of dexamethasone.

Keep in Mind

Unusual behavior in the adolescent cannot be assumed to be related to psychiatric conditions, behavioral disturbance, or drug use.

Not all headaches require imaging or sampling of cerebrospinal fluid, but migraine should be a diagnosis of exclusion, especially in the pediatric emergency setting.

Intracranial abscesses may result from hematogenous spread (as in the case of cyanotic congenital heart disease) or from extension of adjacent infection (as in this case as a complication of paranasal sinus infection).

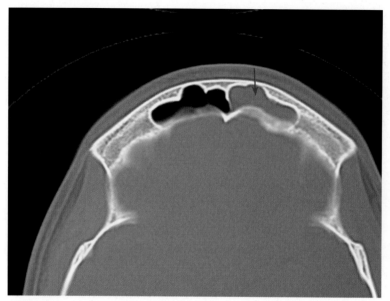

Figure 49-2

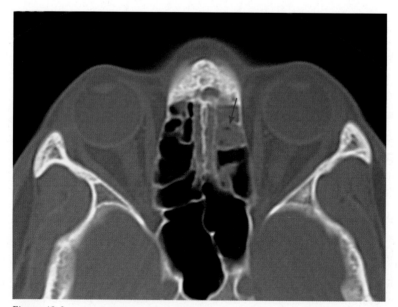

Figure 49-3

The manifestation of intracranial abscesses can be insidious and subtle, or overt and rapidly progressive. Specific symptoms result from the affected region. In the case of epidural abscesses, the adherence of the dura to the skull limits the size of the lesion, and symptoms may be limited to pain and fever. Management combines antibiotic therapy directed at the most likely source of infection, surgical drainage, and close monitoring in a critical care setting.

Recommended Reading

Goodkin HP, Pomeroy SL. Parameningeal infections. In: Feigin RD, Cherry JD, Demmler GJ, Kaplan SL, eds. *Textbook of Pediatric Infectious Diseases.* 5th ed. Philadelphia, PA: WB Saunders; 2004:475–483

Nelson DS. Coma and altered level of consciousness. In: Fleisher GR, Ludwig S, Henretig FM, Ruddy RM, Silverman BK. *Textbook of Pediatric Emergency Medicine.* 5th ed. Philadelphia, PA: Lippincott Williams & Wilkins; 2006:201–212

Chapter 50

Headaches, Fever, and Painful Abdominal Mass

Presentation

A 15-year-old girl seeks care for headache, abdominal pain, and fever of 2 days' duration. The headache is bifrontal in location, and she describes it as throbbing in nature. Ibuprofen affords mild relief. She reports upper abdominal pain without anorexia, nausea, vomiting, or diarrhea. Her temperature rose as high as 39°C, although she reports no fever today. Her mother has noticed a gradual enlargement of the right abdomen over many months. Her relevant medical history includes a midlumbar myelomeningocele and a Chiari malformation with ventriculoperitoneal shunt. The patient has a neurogenic bladder and performs intermittent self-catheterization without assistance. Her last shunt revision was 2 years prior.

She is afebrile with normal vital signs; she is awake and alert in no distress. There is no tenderness, fluctuance, or erythema over the course of the ventriculoperitoneal shunt. Pupils are equally round and reactive to light. There is no nuchal rigidity. A large right upper quadrant mass extends to the level of the umbilicus and is tender to palpation. She has normal strength in the upper extremities and has none in the lower extremities. No jaundice or scleral icterus is present.

Discussion

Differential Diagnosis

- Acquired mass of hepatobiliary, renal, or intestinal origin
- Shunt malfunction (eg, obstruction, disruption, other complication)
- Shunt-related infection
- Urinary infection and complications
- Primary central nervous system infection (eg, meningitis, especially viral; abscess)
- Malignancy

Evaluation

Laboratory studies reveal white blood cells (WBC) 8,900/μL with normal differential, aspartate aminotransferase 78 U/L, alanine aminotransferase 91 U/L, bilirubin 0.2 mg/dL, and alkaline phosphatase 82 U/L. Urinalysis obtained by catheter reveals the presence of nitrites and leukocyte esterase, more than 100 WBC/high-power field, and many bacteria. Cranial computed tomography (CT) scan and shunt series reveal no ventriculomegaly or disruption of the shunt. Abdominal CT reveals a 12 × 16 × 18-cm homogeneous cystic mass in the right abdomen (Figure 50-1) with the shunt tip at the anterior border (Figure 50-2).

Treatment

Although pyuria and bacteriuria may occur during chronic colonization of a neurogenic bladder, the patient also has fever and abdominal symptoms that suggest true infection, and she receives ceftriaxone intravenously while awaiting the results of other studies. However, the abdominal mass is clearly unrelated to urinary infection. Its radiographic appearance and location in relation to the shunt lead you to diagnose a cerebrospinal fluid pseudocyst. The neurosurgery service admits the patient to a monitored ward. During observation, she remains pain free and afebrile. Ultrasound-guided aspiration yields 2 L of clear, acellular fluid with a negative Gram stain. Cyst fluid cultures are negative and the patient recovers, remaining asymptomatic without further intervention. Her urine culture yields growth of *Escherichia coli,* for which she completes outpatient oral antibiotic treatment.

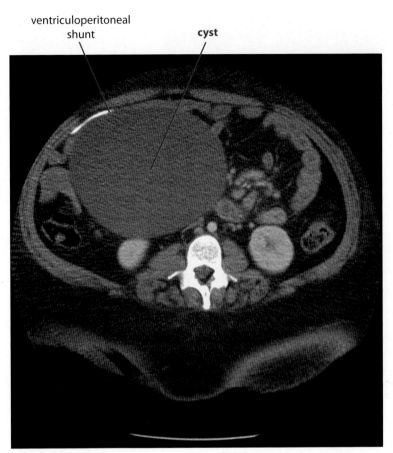

Figure 50-1

Keep in Mind

Abdominal pain in a patient with a ventricular shunt raises the question of shunt complications but often involves diagnoses that may present in otherwise healthy patients without shunts. Headache may result from shunt malfunction or infection.

Urologic pathology and the practice of self-catheterization are risk factors for infection. However, pyuria or bacteriuria in a patient with neurogenic bladder should not dissuade the clinician from pursuing other causes of fever or abdominal symptoms.

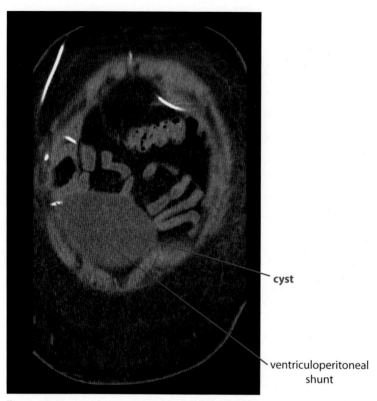

Figure 50-2

Cerebrospinal fluid pseudocyst, an uncommon but well-described complication occurring at the distal end of a ventriculoperitoneal shunt, may
occur with abdominal symptoms or mass, signs of shunt malfunction, or
both. In this case, a component of shunt malfunction may have raised the
intracranial pressure sufficiently to cause headaches without CT evidence
of ventriculomegaly (especially if the patient has poorly compliant ventricles). Signs of infection may or may not be present. Although a mass may
be palpable, CT or ultrasound demonstrating a fluid collection associated
with the catheter confirms the diagnosis. Ultrasound-guided aspiration
will provide relief of local symptoms, exclude or confirm the presence of
infection, and potentially simplify management if elective revision without
externalization is feasible. If no cyst- or shunt-related symptoms recur,

the surgeon may opt to delay or avoid surgery. When infection is present or cannot be excluded with certainty, the shunt may be converted to an external ventricular drain with replacement of the peritoneal catheter after resolution of the cyst.

Recommended Reading

Coley BD, Shiels WE, Elton S, Murakami JW, Hogan MJ. Sonographically guided aspiration of cerebrospinal fluid pseudocysts in children and adolescents. *AJR Am J Roentgenol.* 2004;183:1507–1510

de Oliveira RS, Barbosa A, Vicente A, Machado HR. An alternative approach for management of abdominal cerebrospinal fluid pseudo-cysts in children. *Childs Nerv Syst.* 2007;23:85–90

Roitberg BZ, Tomita T, McLone DG. Abdominal cerebrospinal fluid pseudocyst: a complication of ventriculoperitoneal shunt in children. *Pediatr Neurosurg.* 1998;29:267–273

Chapter 51

Seizure at Grandma's House

Presentation

A 2-year-old boy was noted to have a seizure by his grandmother, who was babysitting over the weekend. The grandmother called an ambulance, which arrived 15 minutes after the call. By this time, the child has stopped seizing. The grandmother describes a generalized seizure that lasted 10 minutes. He now appears drowsy. He is breathing well. He is transported to the emergency department accompanied by his grandparents.

Past medical history is negative.

Examination reveals the following vital signs: temperature 37.4°C, pulse 95 beats/min, respiration 35 breaths/min, blood pressure 95/70 mm Hg, and oxygen saturation 100% in room air. He is drowsy but able to be aroused. Examination of head, eyes, ears, nose, and throat is normal. His neck is supple. His heartbeat is regular with no murmur. His lungs are clear with good aeration. His abdomen is soft and nontender. He moves all his extremities. Tone seems to be diminished. Deep tendon reflexes are 1+ to 2+. Plantar reflexes are upgoing bilaterally. His diaper is saturated with urine.

Discussion

Differential Diagnosis

- Generalized seizure
- Seizure disorder
- Hypoglycemic seizure
- Hyponatremic seizure
- Meningitis
- Encephalitis
- Drug ingestion

Evaluation

Laboratory evaluation is performed with the following findings: sodium 118 mmol/L, potassium 2.8 mmol/L, chloride 90 mmol/L, bicarbonate 29 mmol/L, glucose 130 mg/dL, calcium 9.1 mmol/L, magnesium 2.1 mmol/L, and urine sodium 75 mmol/L. Complete blood count is normal.

The differential diagnosis of hyponatremia includes diuretic ingestion, syndrome of inappropriate antidiuretic hormone (SIADH) (although there is no reason for the patient to have this), salt-losing nephropathy (although there is no history of kidney disease), and adrenal (Addisonian) crisis (no hyperkalemia).

Further history from the grandparents reveals that the grandfather has a history of heart disease. He takes digoxin and a diuretic. The child's digoxin level is checked and is found to be zero. The grandfather thinks that he probably left some of his diuretic pills on a small table, although he is not sure how many. No one is currently at home to inspect the house. A diuretic overdose is suspected.

Treatment

Intravenous normal saline is infused at a modest rate. The patient does well and is discharged after an overnight observation period. On discharge his sodium level was 135 mmol/L.

Keep in Mind

Whenever a child has been in a sitter's home, it should be assumed that the sitter's home is not as childproof as the parents' home. Grandparents often watch children, grandparents often take medication, and grandparents are often not as careful to keep their medications and other objects out of the reach of children.

When children swallow pills or ingest a substance, the quantity swallowed is frequently unknown. The event is rarely witnessed by an adult because if it was witnessed, it would have been stopped. Thus, the severity of the ingestion is almost never known.

Hyponatremia is a known cause of seizures; however, sodium values low enough to cause a seizure are not common.

The identification of significant hyponatremia should be immediately followed by a measurement of the urine sodium. If the child's physiology is normal, hyponatremia should only occur in conjunction with a low urine sodium because the kidneys should be trying to retain sodium. High urine sodium, as in this case, limits the causes of hyponatremia to diuretic effects, SIADH, salt-losing nephropathy, and adrenal crisis (Addisonian salt-losing crisis).

Most diuretics stimulate sodium excretion even in the face of total body sodium depletion. Hyponatremia resulting from diuretics is best treated by stopping the diuretics and administering normal saline.

Syndrome of inappropriate antidiuretic hormone usually occurs in conjunction with severe debilitating conditions such as bacterial meningitis, severe brain conditions, or severe systemic disease. Antidiuretic hormone–like hormones are released, which causes fluid retention and inappropriate sodium excretion, resulting in hyponatremia. The treatment for SIADH is fluid restriction.

A salt-losing nephropathy is associated with renal disease in which dysfunctioning kidneys are unable to retain sodium appropriately, resulting in hyponatremia. Sodium replacement is necessary in most instances.

In adrenal crisis, a lack of mineralocorticoids results in sodium excretion and potassium retention. Concurrent glucocorticoid deficiency can result in hypoglycemia and multisystem failure and shock. Congenital adrenal hyperplasia (21-hydroxylase deficiency) is the most common cause in young infants. Withdrawal from long-term corticosteroid therapy (eg, to treat Crohn disease or collagen vascular disease) with insufficient corticosteroid replacement therapy is another cause.

Chapter 52

Seizure After a Swimming Lesson

Presentation

A 15-month-old male was being driven home from a swimming lesson at a swim club. His mother happened to look in her rearview mirror, and she saw her child's head jerking. She stopped the car and noted that her child was seizing with his eyes deviated superiorly. She called 911 on her mobile phone, and an ambulance shortly arrived. By this time, the child had stopped seizing. She described a 10-minute generalized seizure to the paramedics. The child appeared drowsy. He was breathing well and had good color. He was transported to the emergency department.

Past medical history is negative.

Examination reveals the following vital signs: rectal temperature 37.2°C, pulse 95 beats/min, respiration 35 breaths/min, blood pressure 110/70 mm Hg, and oxygen saturation 99% in room air. He is drowsy but able to be aroused. Examination of head, eyes, ears, nose, and throat is normal. His neck is supple. His heartbeat is regular with no murmur. His lungs are clear with good aeration. His abdomen is soft and non-tender. He has slight hypotonia. Deep tendon reflexes are 1+ to 2+. Plantar reflexes are upgoing bilaterally. Skin is well perfused with no lesions.

Discussion

Differential Diagnosis

- Generalized seizure
- Seizure disorder
- Hypoglycemic seizure
- Hyponatremic seizure
- Meningitis

Evaluation

Laboratory evaluation is performed with the following findings: bedside glucose 130 mg/dL, sodium 121 mmol/L, potassium 3.5 mmol/L, chloride 94 mmol/L, bicarbonate 20 mmol/L, glucose 130 mg/dL, calcium 9.1 mmol/L, magnesium 2.1 mmol/L, and urine sodium 50 mmol/L. Complete blood count is performed, with the following findings: white blood cells 18,100/μL, 60% segmented neutrophils, 5% bands, 35% lymphocytes, hemoglobin 13 g/dL, hematocrit 39%, and platelet count 400,000/μL.

The patient is diagnosed with hyponatremic seizure and water intoxication.

Treatment

The treatment for symptomatic hyponatremia is hypertonic saline administration. However, the use of hypertonic saline is potentially risky. More conservative treatments are fluid restriction, normal saline administration, and free-water diuretics (eg, mannitol). The treatment of symptomatic hyponatremia is beyond the scope of this chapter.

Keep in Mind

In the 1970s and 1980s, infant swimming lessons were popular. Television documentaries showed infants happily swimming underwater with their eyes open. These babies appeared to be comfortable in the water.

However, while these infants were happily swimming, many of them were swallowing lots of water. Diarrhea and polyuria were common after an infant swim lesson. Some infants became water intoxicated and developed seizures. Many reports of hyponatremic seizures associated with infant swimming lessons led to this practice being discouraged.

Providing swimming lessons to young children might give parents a false sense of security about water safety. Even if a young child can swim in a pool, young children still lack the skills to assess environmental risk. Rough surf, strong currents, slippery rocks, and situations that require more advanced water survival skills will overwhelm many children who are capable of swimming in a supervised pool environment.

Children are generally not developmentally ready for formal swimming lessons until after their fourth birthday. Aquatic programs for infants and toddlers should not be promoted as a way to decrease the risk of drowning. Parents should not feel secure that their child is safe in water or safe from drowning after their children have participated in such programs. Whenever infants and toddlers are in or around water, an adult should be within an arm's length, providing touch supervision.

Recommended Reading

American Academy of Pediatrics, Committee on Sports Medicine and Fitness and Committee on Injury and Poison Prevention. Swimming programs for infants and toddlers. *Pediatrics.* 2000;105:868–870

Chapter 53

Seizures 1

Presentation

An 18-month-old girl experiences onset of generalized seizures. She
had been vomiting since the morning and she has a fever (temperature
up to 38.5°C). An ambulance is called, which arrives 20 minutes later.
They find the child to have generalized seizures with facial cyanosis. An
attempt to place an intravenous (IV) line is not successful. Glucose check
is 130 mg/dL. They call the emergency department (ED) on the radio and
ask for further instructions. Rectal diazepam is ordered and administered.
The patient is transported. While in transit, a second IV attempt is successful, and IV diazepam is administered. The seizure becomes less intense for
about 3 minutes, but then returns to the same state of generalized tonic-
clonic seizures. They arrive at the ED with the patient still seizing. Color
is pink with blow-by oxygen.

Past medical history is negative.

Examination reveals the following vital signs: axillary temperature 37.3°C,
heart rate by electrocardiogram 130 beats/min (sinus tachycardia), and
respiratory rate difficult to count because of seizures. Blood pressure is not
obtainable, even after several attempts. Oxygen saturation is 100% on supplemental oxygen by mask. The patient exhibits generalized seizure activity
with eyes rolled up and body jerking. Pupils are small. Tympanic membranes are normal. Her mouth is difficult to examine, as is her neck muscle
tone. Her heartbeat is regular with no murmurs. Her lungs exhibit shallow
aeration. An examination of her abdomen is difficult to perform. Neurologic examination is limited by the generalized tonic-clonic seizures.

Discussion

Differential Diagnosis

- New-onset seizure disorder
- Epilepsy
- Status epilepticus (SE)
- Metabolic seizure
- Meningitis
- Encephalitis
- Brain hemorrhage
- Brain lesion
- Drug ingestion

Evaluation

Laboratory evaluation reveals the following findings: bedside glucose 150 mg/dL, sodium 134 mmol/L, potassium 3.1 mmol/L, chloride 99 mmol/L, bicarbonate 22 mmol/L, glucose 161 mg/dL, and calcium 10.0 mg/dL.

Complete blood count is performed with the following findings: white blood cells 22,200/μL, 60% segmented neutrophils, 10% bands, 30% lymphocytes, hemoglobin 13 g/dL, hematocrit 39%, and platelet count 470,000/μL.

Treatment

Rectal and IV diazepam have been given by paramedics en route. Seizure intensity declined briefly, but the seizures started again. An IV dose of lorazepam 0.1 mg/kg is administered in the ED. After 4 minutes, no improvement is noted. A second dose of lorazepam 0.1 mg/kg is administered. Fosphenytoin 15 mg/kg is given IV. Seizures continue, so phenobarbital 15 mg/kg is given IV. A time sequence of events is listed in Table 53-1.

A lumbar puncture is performed after the CT. Initial opening pressure is 15 cm H_2O (normal). Analysis of the cerebrospinal fluid reveals the following: 90 red blood cells/μL, 40 white blood cells/μL, 50% segmented neutrophils, 50% monocytes, total protein 59 g/dL, and glucose 70 mg/dL. Gram stain reveals few white blood cells, but no organisms are seen. Herpes polymerase chain reaction is positive.

Table 53-1. Time Sequence of Events in Patient With Generalized Seizures

Time	Event
10:00	Seizure starts.
10:02	Parents call 911.
10:20	Paramedics arrive at home.
10:23	Paramedics enter home and witness seizures.
10:24	Oxygen mask applied.
10:25	Electrocardiogram leads placed.
10:27	Intravenous (IV) access attempted but unsuccessful.
10:29	Rectal diazepam administered.
10:33	Patient bundled onto gurney and moved into ambulance.
10:35	Transport begins.
10:38	Second IV attempt is successful.
10:41	IV diazepam is given.
10:45	Seizures severity subsides briefly.
10:48	Seizure severity returns.
10:57	Ambulance arrives at hospital.
10:59	Patient is now on a gurney in the ED.
11:00	Blood is drawn for laboratory tests.
11:03	Lorazepam 0.1 mg/kg is given IV.
11:07	Second lorazepam dose 0.1 mg/kg is given IV.
11:08	Fosphenytoin 15 mg/kg is given slowly IV.
11:15	Fosphenytoin infusion completed.
11:23	Phenobarbital 15 mg/kg is given slowly IV.
11:28	Phenobarbital infusion completed.
11:30	Rapid sequence intubation is initiated.
11:33	Intubation is confirmed via end-tidal P_{CO_2}.
11:36	IV antibiotics are pushed.
11:38	IV acyclovir infusion is started.
11:47	A computed tomography scan of the brain is completed.

You diagnose the patient with prolonged refractory SE due to herpes encephalitis.

The computed tomography (CT) scan shown in Figure 53-1 was taken from a different patient with herpes encephalitis; it shows bilateral temporal lobe abnormalities. Most initial CT scans of patients with encephalitis are not as dramatic.

One hour and 28 minutes has elapsed from the onset of the seizure to the completion of the phenobarbital infusion, and the seizures still have not stopped. The approach described herein can be called the give-and-check approach, in which a drug is provided and the status of the seizures are reassessed a few minutes later. If a reasonable period to assess the efficacy of an anticonvulsant is roughly 3 to 5 minutes, this process could continue for a long time.

In SE, the patient's brain is hypermetabolic, demanding more glucose and oxygen substrates, yet the generalized seizures result in shallow respirations and hypoxia. High-flow supplemental oxygen can usually normalize oxygenation, but respiratory acidosis from hypercarbia is often present. Brief seizures are not associated with brain injury, whereas prolonged seizures place the patient at risk of hypoxic brain injury. The goal in treating SE is to stop the seizures as soon as possible and to optimize oxygen delivery.

Status epilepticus can be categorized into simple SE and refractory SE. In simple SE, the seizures terminate after 1 or 2 doses of a benzodiazepine

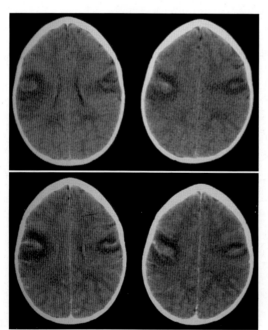

Figure 53-1

(eg, diazepam, lorazepam, midazolam). In refractory SE, seizures continue despite several benzodiazepine doses and other IV anticonvulsants such as phenytoin (or fosphenytoin) and phenobarbital. Encephalitis can manifest as simple SE, but it often manifests as refractory SE. Failure to stop the seizures after 1 or 2 benzodiazepine doses suggests the possibility of refractory SE.

If IV access is not available, rectal diazepam is an option. The dose should be at least doubled if it is given rectally because absorption is unpredictable. Intramuscular (IM) midazolam is also an option. If IV access is established after rectal diazepam or IM midazolam administration, another benzodiazepine dose should be provided IV because rectal or IM drug absorption is less reliable.

A therapeutic controversy that arises in the management of refractory SE is how soon to paralyze and intubate the patient by using rapid sequence intubation (RSI). Early RSI makes sense. With RSI, the patient's airway is controlled, oxygen delivery is optimized, Pco_2 is normalized, pH is normalized, muscle activity is reduced, and most importantly, maximal doses of anticonvulsants can be provided because the potential for apnea is inconsequential. Rapid sequence intubation also facilitates CT scanning and performing a lumbar puncture. The major concern of RSI that causes clinicians to hesitate is that if brain seizure activity is still present, we cannot witness the seizure activity. Once RSI is initiated, we should assume that the brain seizure activity is persisting and maximal anticonvulsant therapy should be administered. Electroencephalogram monitoring in the ED is a theoretical possibility, but few medical centers are able to implement this. Thiopental, provided as part of RSI, is also a potent anticonvulsant. Maximum loading doses of phenytoin and phenobarbital should be administered. The role of other, newer IV anticonvulsants such as valproic acid and levetiracetam is unclear.

In this particular case, compare the therapeutic management using the give-and-check approach versus an early RSI approach. In the give-and-check approach, one has to wait to determine the clinical effect of each drug. In the early RSI approach, we assume that seizure activity is ongoing and all drugs are provided as rapidly as possible. This facilitates giving the most anticonvulsant drug therapy in the shortest possible time.

Keep in Mind

If you believe that RSI results in a better set of clinical circumstances in the management of refractory SE, RSI should be initiated once refractory SE becomes a possibility. Failure to terminate the seizures with 2 benzodiazepine doses allows you to classify the patient as being at risk of refractory SE.

Status epilepticus can be the first symptom of encephalitis. Most of the encephalitis viruses cannot be treated, but herpes encephalitis can be treated with acyclovir. Early treatment is likely to be better than late treatment; therefore, administering IV acyclovir empirically as part of the early ED drug management of such patients is potentially beneficial.

Recommended Reading

Chiang VW. Seizures. In: Fleisher GR, Ludwig S, Henretig FM, Ruddy RM, Silverman BK, eds. *Textbook of Pediatric Emergency Medicine.* 5th ed. Philadelphia, PA: Lippincott Williams & Wilkins; 2006:629–636

Farooq MU, Naravetla B, Majid A, et al. IV levetiracetam in the management of non-convulsive status epilepticus. *Neurocrit Care.* 2007;7:36–39

Gorelick MH, Blackwell CD. Neurologic emergencies. In: Fleisher GR, Ludwig S, Henretig FM, Ruddy RM, Silverman BK, eds. *Textbook of Pediatric Emergency Medicine.* 5th ed. Philadelphia, PA: Lippincott Williams & Wilkins; 2006:759–781

Isaacman DJ, Trainor JL, Rothrock SG. Central nervous system. In: Gausche-Hill M, Fuchs S, Yamamoto L, eds. *APLS: The Pediatric Emergency Medicine Resource.* 4th rev ed. Sudbury, MA: Jones and Bartlett Publishers; 2007:146–185

Marr JK. Encephalitis. In: Yamamoto LG, Inaba AS, Okamoto JK, Patronis ME, Yamashiroya VK, eds. *Case Based Pediatrics for Medical Students and Residents.* Honolulu, HI: University of Hawaii; 2004:189–193. Available at: http://www.hawaii.edu/medicine/pediatrics/pedtext. Accessed December 30, 2008

Yamamoto LG. Emergency airway management—rapid sequence intubation. In: Fleisher GR, Ludwig S, Henretig FM, Ruddy RM, Silverman BK, eds. *Textbook of Pediatric Emergency Medicine.* 5th ed. Philadelphia, PA: Lippincott Williams & Wilkins; 2006:81–92

Yamamoto LG. Status epilepticus. In: Yamamoto LG, Inaba AS, Okamoto JK, Patronis ME, Yamashiroya VK, eds. *Case Based Pediatrics for Medical Students and Residents.* Honolulu, HI: University of Hawaii; 2004:547–549. Available at: http://www.hawaii.edu/medicine/pediatrics/pedtext. Accessed December 30, 2008

Yamamoto LG, Yim GK. The role of intravenous valproic acid in status epilepticus. *Pediatr Emerg Care.* 2000;16:296–298

Chapter 54

Seizures 2

Presentation

A 17-year-old girl experiences onset of generalized seizures. Her mother did not know that her daughter was ill until she heard some noises in her daughter's room and went to check on her. She found her daughter's body stiff and jerking, with her eyes rolled up. She was drooling and blue in the face. Her mother called 911 and paramedics quickly arrived. She was placed on oxygen, an intravenous (IV) line was started, and IV diazepam was administered. She arrived in the emergency department (ED) a short time later, still seizing.

Past medical history is reportedly negative. The mother does not know the date of her daughter's last menstrual period.

Examination reveals the following vital signs: axillary temperature 36.7°C, heart rate on electrocardiogram 90 beats/min (sinus tachycardia), and respiratory rate difficult to count because of seizures. Her blood pressure is not obtainable, even after several attempts. Oxygen saturation is 100% on supplemental oxygen by nonrebreather mask. She exhibits generalized seizure activity, with her eyes superiorly deviated and her body jerking. Her pupils are small. Her tympanic membranes are normal. Her mouth is difficult to examine. Neck muscle tone is difficult to examine. Her heartbeat is regular with no murmurs. Her lungs have shallow aeration. Her abdominal contour is normal. Neurologic examination is limited by generalized tonic-clonic seizures. Perfusion is good.

Discussion

Differential Diagnosis

- New-onset seizure disorder
- Epilepsy
- Status epilepticus
- Drug overdose
- Meningitis
- Encephalitis
- Brain hemorrhage or lesion

Evaluation

Laboratory evaluation is performed, and bedside glucose is found to be 150 mg/dL.

Intravenous lorazepam is administered and repeated 2 minutes later. Blood samples are drawn and sent to the laboratory for study. The seizures continue. Refractory status epilepticus is suspected. The patient is intubated by rapid sequence intubation (RSI). Drugs used include thiopental and rocuronium. Visible seizure activity stops. She is treated with 20 mg/kg of IV fosphenytoin and 20 mg/kg of IV phenobarbital as well as IV antibiotics and IV acyclovir. She is catheterized so a urine sample can be obtained. A urine human chorionic gonadotropin study is negative. The urine is sent for a stat drug screen. A computed tomography (CT) scan of the brain shows no abnormalities.

The mother brought her daughter's purse with her. Although the mother initially indicated that her daughter's past medical history is negative, she now discloses that her daughter has been taking isoniazid (INH) for the past 3 months. The nurse finds the INH pill bottle in the purse. The bottle has a few pills remaining, and from the date of the prescription, it's clear that there should be more pills in the bottle. Her mother is asked whether there is any chance that her daughter might have overdosed on these pills, whether there has been any major stress recently, or whether any sign of depression has been evident. The mother replies with an emphatic "no," even when the questions are repeated. The ED physician suspects the worst-case scenario: this could be an INH overdose.

Treatment

A toxicology reference reveals that the treatment for INH overdose resulting in seizures is pyridoxine. The dose is 5,000 mg IV, which is ordered emergently. The night-shift pharmacist calls the ED physician to verify the extremely high dose of pyridoxine. The physician and pharmacist discuss the indication for the high dose of pyridoxine and concur that 5,000 mg is the proper dose. Intravenous pyridoxine comes in 100-mg vials, and the dose is 5,000 mg, so 50 vials are required. However, the pharmacy has only 10 vials. Larger vial sizes are available, but these are typically carried by poison centers. The pharmacist calls 3 other hospital pharmacies nearby, requesting assistance. These hospital pharmacies send their pyridoxine ampules to the ED, where the full dose is administered.

The patient's urine drug screening results are negative. She is transferred to the intensive care unit. Her serum INH level subsequently returns as very high. She recovers well, and she later discloses that she deliberately overdosed on the INH because she was under a great deal of stress and wanted to kill herself.

Keep in Mind

This patient presents with refractory status epilepticus, as evidenced by failure to terminate the seizures with 2 doses of lorazepam. The therapeutic option of early RSI was exercised in this case to secure her airway, optimize oxygen delivery, normalize her P_{CO_2}, maximize anticonvulsant drug dosing, and facilitate CT scanning.

Teen suicide gestures are not uncommon. Most of the time, the overdose is with a drug that the teen has easy access to. Acetaminophen overdose is common and can be lethal, but in most instances, the overdose is not toxic or the patient seeks treatment early. Teens with access to large quantities of chronic medications such as anticonvulsants, cardiac medications, and psychotropic medications can easily intentionally overdose on drugs. An INH ingestion is uncommon in adolescents. Some teens have access to large quantities of INH because of tuberculosis exposure prophylaxis.

Pyridoxine treatment is an effective antidote, but because the dose required is extremely large, many hospitals do not have a sufficient stock of IV pyridoxine. This is true of many antidotes. Digoxin-binding antibody fragments and snake antivenom are examples of antidotes that are needed rarely, but when the need arises, it is urgent. Hospitals in communities should form partnerships to share stocks of drugs that are uncommonly used. In this case, hospital pharmacies in the community had prearranged agreements for this type of drug sharing, making the full dose of the pyridoxine antidote readily available. Rural hospitals in isolated areas have a more difficult problem with ensuring availability of antidotes.

Recommended Reading

Chiang VW. Seizures. In: Fleisher GR, Ludwig S, Henretig FM, Ruddy RM, Silverman BK, eds. *Textbook of Pediatric Emergency Medicine.* 5th ed. Philadelphia, PA: Lippincott Williams & Wilkins; 2006:629–636

Isoniazid. Poisindex summary. In: *Micromedex Healthcare Series* [intranet database]. Version 5.1. Greenwood Village, CO: Thomson Healthcare; 2008

Chapter 55

Seizures 3

Presentation

A 2-month-old boy with a history of a ventricular septal defect (VSD) arrives in the emergency department (ED) for a possible seizure. This evening, his parents noted an episode of body stiffness, jerking of all extremities, and upward rolling of his eyes lasting 1 minute. His face was described as being blue toward the end of the episode. Paramedics noted him to be breathing spontaneously with no cyanosis. He was transported to the ED. There was no recent history of fever or head trauma.

Past medical history indicates that he was born at term and had normal Apgar scores. In the nursery, he was noted to have a heart murmur. A chest radiograph showed mild cardiomegaly. An echocardiogram confirmed this to be a VSD with a mild degree of congestive heart failure. He is currently under the care of a cardiologist and is being treated with digoxin.

Your examination reveals the following vital signs: rectal temperature 36.6°C, pulse 132 beats/min, respiration 60 breaths/min, and oxygen saturation 98% in room air. The patient is alert and active. His anterior fontanelle is soft and flat. His neck is supple. His heartbeat is regular with a harsh grade 3/6 systolic murmur. His lungs are clear and he has good color, perfusion, and tone.

Shortly after arrival in the ED, another seizure occurs, which is witnessed by the ED staff. His upper extremities are flexed and jerking. His lower extremities are extended and jerking. No one recalls what his eyes were doing. An intravenous (IV) line is attempted during the seizure but is unsuccessful. The seizure stops spontaneously after 5 minutes. His oxygen saturation is 100% throughout the seizure with an oxygen mask in place. After the seizure, he is crying and does not appear drowsy. He moves all

4 extremities during attempts to place an IV line. He is noted to be very strong. An IV is finally started, and he is given 0.1 mg/kg of lorazepam and 10 mg/kg of phenobarbital, which appear to sedate him. His respiratory effort and perfusion remain good.

Discussion

Differential Diagnosis
- New-onset seizure disorder
- Brain infarction with history of VSD
- Metabolic abnormality

Evaluation
Laboratory evaluations are performed with the following results: sodium 133 mmol/L, potassium 4.4 mmol/L, chloride 91 mmol/L, bicarbonate 26 mmol/L, glucose 144 mg/dL, creatinine 0.4 mg/dL, calcium 6.0 mg/dL (normal range, 8.0–10.0 mg/dL), digoxin level within the therapeutic range, magnesium 1.9 mEq/L, and phosphate 8.9 mg/dL (normal range, 4.0–6.0 mg/dL). Complete blood count is normal.

Chest radiographs are ordered.

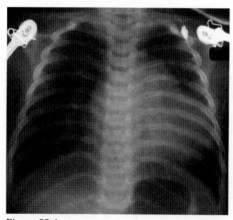

Figure 55-1

The patient's anteroposterior (AP) and lateral chest radiographs are displayed in figures 55-1 and 55-2. Cardiomegaly is evident, but the lungs are clear. The specific abnormality noted is the absence of a thymic shadow. The AP view shows a very narrow mediastinum. The lateral view shows air density lung tissue in the anterior mediastinum (anterior to the heart).

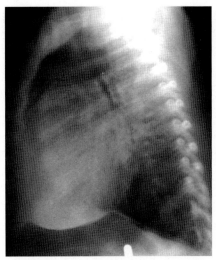

Figure 55-2

The 2 AP chest radiographs in Figure 55-3 are from healthy neonates. There is a prominent thymic shadow, which is normal in this age group—and very different from the chest radiograph of our patient.

The lateral chest radiograph in Figure 55-4 shows a normal thymus in the anterior mediastinum. The tiny black arrows point to this region, which should normally be filled with a tissue density in young infants. As the size of the thymus decreases, this space should be filled with lung (air density). In our patient's lateral chest radiograph view, there is no thymic tissue density in the anterior mediastinum.

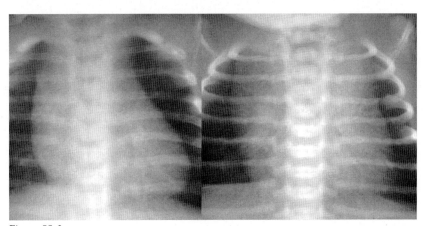

Figure 55-3

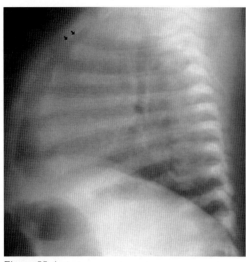

Figure 55-4

Treatment
The patient is hospitalized and an endocrinologist is consulted to correct the hypocalcemia due to suspected hypoparathyroidism. You diagnose the child with DiGeorge syndrome.

Keep in Mind
The patient's chest radiograph and the hypocalcemia confirm the presence of thymic aplasia (T-cell deficiency) and hypoparathyroidism (hypocalcemia), diagnostic of DiGeorge syndrome. DiGeorge syndrome is also associated with facial anomalies and cardiac malformations. DiGeorge syndrome is more commonly included in the group of congenital immuno-deficiency syndromes. However, patients with DiGeorge syndrome will manifest symptoms at a very young age with hypocalcemia, generally long before they experience opportunistic infection.

Recommended Reading
Yamamoto LG. Seizure and VSD in 2-month-old infant. In: Yamamoto LG, Inaba AS, DiMauro R, eds. *Radiology Cases in Pediatric Emergency Medicine*. Vol 2, case 2. March 1995. Available at: http://www.hawaii.edu/medicine/pediatrics/pemxray/v2c02.html. Accessed December 30, 2008

Part 6

Head and Neck Presentations

Chapter 56

Jaw Swelling

Presentation

A 7-year-old boy is brought to the emergency department (ED) because of jaw swelling and pain that is most notable in both cheeks. The swelling on his left is greater than the right. He has no history of fever. His parents noticed the swelling in the evening. His pain increased and the swelling was so prominent that they called his primary care physician, who advised them to bring him to the ED. He has no cough, vomiting, or diarrhea. He ate dinner normally. His past medical history is unremarkable. He is fully immunized and his mother specifically remembers that he received 2 measles, mumps, and rubella immunizations.

Examination reveals the following: oral temperature 37.2°C, pulse 97 beats/min, respiration 20 breaths/min, blood pressure 90/65 mm Hg, and oxygen saturation 99% in room air. He is alert and cooperative, but moderately uncomfortable as a result of pain. His eyes show clear conjunctiva. Tympanic membranes are normal. His nose and pharynx are clear. His oral mucosa is moist. The Stensen ducts are visible on both sides, but are only slightly prominent. No pus is visible draining from the duct. He has prominent bilateral swellings over his mandibular angles (Figure 56-1). The swelling is firm and moderately tender. No redness is evident. No other discrete swellings can be palpated in his lower neck. His neck range of motion is good. Heart and lungs are normal. His abdomen is nontender with no hepatosplenomegaly or masses. No inguinal hernias are visible. His scrotum shows no redness or swelling. His testes are nontender. His extremities are normal. His color and perfusion are good.

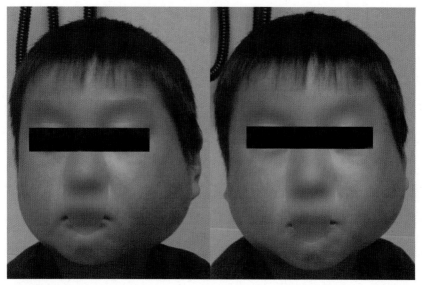

Figure 56-1

Discussion

Differential Diagnosis
- Parotitis
- Mumps

Evaluation
Mumps is unlikely because he is fully immunized, he has not traveled out of the country, and the community is not currently experiencing a mumps epidemic. Other viral causes of parotitis are more likely. Bacterial parotitis is not likely because it is bilateral. A parotid calculus is likewise unlikely, again because it is bilateral, although it is possible that a calculus could subsequently develop as a complication of the parotitis. Although lymph-adenopathy is possible, whenever the swelling crosses the upslope of the mandibular angle, parotitis is the likely cause.

The final diagnosis is parotitis.

Treatment

Acetaminophen with hydrocodone is provided for pain control. Twenty minutes later, the patient is smiling and much more comfortable. He is discharged home.

His immunization history is confirmed, and his parents are advised to monitor his scrotum by checking for any swelling. The option of obtaining mumps antibody titers is offered but declined by his parents. He is prescribed analgesics and cephalexin as prophylaxis against bacterial overgrowth and calculus formation. These measures are probably not necessary but make the doctor feel more comfortable. His parents are advised not to mention or present foods to him that will promote excess saliva flow, such as lemons, pickles, or salty snacks, because these can cause severe parotid pain in some patients.

During follow-up, his parotid swelling subsides, and he returns to his normal state of health in a few days.

Keep in Mind

Mumps is caused by an RNA paramyxovirus. Mumps is uncommon today because of widespread immunization. This patient was fully immunized in a community with a high immunization rate and no known outbreak of mumps.

Other reported viral causes of parotitis include HIV infection, influenza, parainfluenza virus, cytomegalovirus, and coxsackieviruses. Bacterial parotitis due to *Staphylococcus aureus* is associated with visible pus that can be expressed through the Stensen duct. Salivary calculi, uncommon in children, can cause parotitis or theoretically result from the inflammatory process. Orchitis (testicular inflammation) and oophoritis (ovarian inflammation) have been described with mumps parotitis and less commonly with other causes of parotitis.

There is no specific therapy except for analgesics. Some have recommended avoiding foods that promote excess salivary flow.

Recommended Reading

Maldonado Y. Mumps. In: Kliegman RM, Behrman RE, Jenson HB, Stanton BF, eds. *Nelson Textbook of Pediatrics.* 18th ed. Int ed. Philadelphia, PA: WB Saunders; 2007:1341–1344

Chapter 57

Neck and Back Pain With Fever

Presentation

A previously healthy 6-year-old boy presents at the emergency department (ED) with 2 days of neck and back pain and fevers as high as 39.7°C. He has mild abdominal pain and has vomited several times, but otherwise he tolerates liquids. He complains of headaches, which he has had for 2 days. He experienced back pain 2 or 3 weeks before after playing a soccer game, but he denies direct trauma. His parents noticed no photophobia, neck rigidity, sore throat, red eyes, diarrhea, joint pain, or rash.

Other than moderate tachycardia (pulse 146 beats/min), his vital signs are normal (respiratory rate 24 breaths/min, blood pressure 104/64 mm Hg), and his oxyhemoglobin saturation is 99% in room air. He is alert and well perfused. Lungs are clear to auscultation with no wheezing, rhonchi, rales, or retractions. His abdomen is soft and nontender with no hepatosplenomegaly. The lower cervical spine and upper thoracic spine are mildly tender. The neck and back demonstrate a full range of motion. Normal tone and strength are present with no meningismus. No rash is present.

Discussion

Differential Diagnosis
- Meningitis
- Diskitis
- Osteomyelitis
- Epidural abscess
- Musculoskeletal injury
- Urinary tract infection or nephrolithiasis with infection

Evaluation
This patient sought care for neck and back pain, headache, fevers, and vomiting. Although meningitis is the most worrisome possibility, you think that the level of alertness and lack of meningeal signs make a central nervous system infection unlikely.

You order screening laboratory tests, but they provide no reassurance. His high white blood cell count (28,300/μL with 76% neutrophils, 12% band forms, and 12% lymphocytes) and erythrocyte sedimentation rate (ESR) (66 mm/h) suggest significant systemic inflammation but do little to narrow the diagnostic list. A rapid streptococcal antigen test is negative. Dipstick urinalysis reveals no blood, nitrites, or leukocyte esterase. Radiographs of the cervical and thoracic spine (figures 57-1 and 57-2) reveal normal bony architecture. Closer inspection of the thoracic study suggests loss of definition of the left hemidiaphragm. A subsequent chest radiograph confirms the presence of an infiltrate in the left lower lobe (figures 57-3 and 57-4). You diagnose the boy with occult pneumonia.

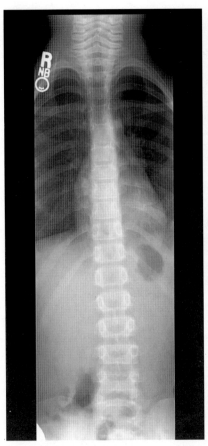

Figure 57-1

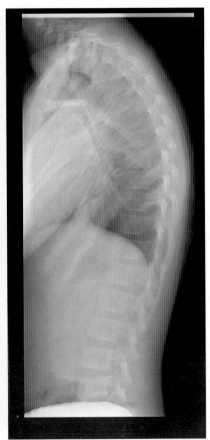

Figure 57-2

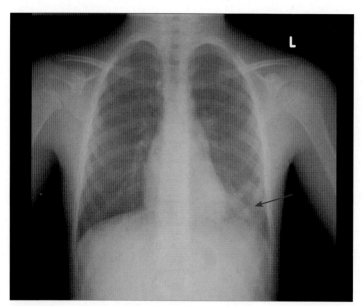

Figure 57-3

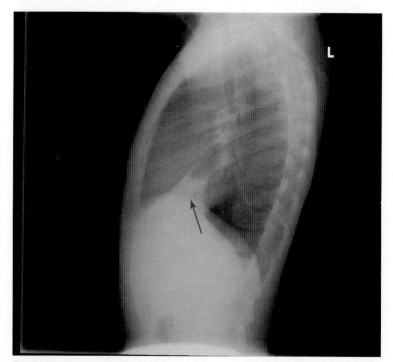

Figure 57-4

Treatment

The patient is provided ceftriaxone 50 mg/kg intramuscularly and a 10-day course of amoxicillin (90 mg/kg/day).

Keep in Mind

Severe neck and back pain in the young should be investigated aggressively, especially when accompanied by fever. The evaluation often involves spinal radiography and laboratory evaluation for evidence of inflammation. Radiographic studies outside of the axial skeleton are rarely conducted. However, this case illustrates the importance of studying the entire radiograph to identify unexpected diagnostic findings.

Serious underlying pathology is found in approximately half of children referred for orthopedic evaluation of back pain. In the pediatric ED, less serious and nonspecific diagnoses such as musculoskeletal pain occur in just under half. Categories of pathology intrinsic to the vertebral column include mechanical (herniation), developmental (spondylolysis, spondylolisthesis, and Scheuermann kyphosis), inflammatory and infectious (diskitis and osteomyelitis), and neoplastic. Extrinsic causes include retrocecal appendicitis, pyelonephritis, hydronephrosis, psoas abscess, and intraabdominal and retroperitoneal masses or neoplasm. Psychosomatic diagnoses should only be considered after organic pathology has been excluded. Children younger than 10 years are more likely to have infectious or neoplastic causes for their back pain, whereas those older than 10 years are more likely to be experiencing developmental or mechanical disorders.

Pneumonia occasionally has an atypical manifestation; it may appear as pain in unusual locations (back or abdomen) or, rarely, as fever in the absence of suggestive respiratory symptoms. Fever is usually present with bacterial disease. Pneumonia mimics an acute abdomen through referred pain, and a similar process may occur in the case of pneumonia causing back pain.

The diagnosis of pneumonia in the febrile child is complicated by a lack of reliable clinical and laboratory predictors. The classic triad of fever, cough, and rales is not always reliable. In some cases, persistent fever may be the only reliable finding. Among children with proven pneumonia, leukocyte counts of greater than 15,000/μL and positive C-reactive protein tests predict the response to antibiotic therapy and a lobar distribution of the infiltrate. In children with fever, an ESR of greater than or equal to 30 mm/h often implies the presence of a bacterial infection, including pneumonia. Among children with fever and no obvious focus of infection, a leukocyte count of greater than or equal to 20,000/μL may suggest an occult pneumonia.

Atypical presentations of common conditions are more likely than unusual conditions.

Recommended Reading

Bachur R, Perry H, Harper MB. Occult pneumonias: empiric chest radiographs in febrile children with leukocytosis. *Ann Emerg Med.* 1999;33:166–173

Kanegaye JT, Harley JR. Pneumonia in unexpected locations: an occult cause of pediatric abdominal pain. *J Emerg Med.* 1995;13:773–779

Murphy CG, Vandepol AC, Harper MB, et al. Clinical predictors of occult pneumonia in the febrile child. *Acad Emerg Med.* 2007;14:243–249

Yee VK, Kanegaye JT. Back pain and fever. *Clin Pediatr.* 2003;42:749–751

Chapter 58

Throat and Neck Pain

Presentation

An 8-year-old boy is brought to the emergency department because of
a sore throat and increasing neck swelling. His symptoms began in the
morning and it is now the evening. He has had a fever, but his temperature
was not measured at home. His appetite is fair but clearly less than usual.
He has a slight cough. His urine output is good. There is no vomiting
or diarrhea.

Past medical, social, and family histories are not contributory.

Examination reveals the following vital signs: oral temperature 39.3°C,
pulse 97 beats/min, respiration 20 breaths/min, blood pressure 90/65 mm
Hg, and oxygen saturation 99% in room air. He is alert and cooperative.
His voice is not hoarse and there is no drooling. His conjunctiva are clear,
his tympanic membranes are normal, and his nose is clear. His pharynx
appears visibly normal. His oral mucosa is moist. His tongue is normal
and without elevation, nor is there induration of the floor of his mouth.
His neck is supple, but he has bilateral tenderness and diffuse swelling
over most of his anterior neck. Some redness is noted. Heart and lungs
are normal. His abdomen is nontender with no hepatosplenomegaly or
masses. His extremities are normal. His color and perfusion are good.

Discussion

Differential Diagnosis
- Viral pharyngitis
- Streptococcal pharyngitis
- Lymphadenitis
- Cellulitis
- Ludwig angina

Evaluation
A swab from the patient's pharynx is obtained and sent for a rapid strep-tococcal test, which returns negative. At this point, the nurse and resident notice that the patient's neck swelling has visibly increased. His mother agrees. His swelling and redness are now quite impressive (Figure 58-1). A lateral neck radiograph and a chest radiograph are obtained to confirm that he does not have a retropharyngeal abscess or a mediastinal abscess. Both are negative.

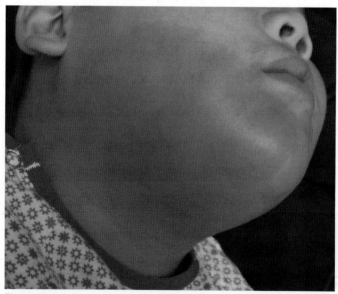

Figure 58-1

An intravenous (IV) line is started, blood is drawn for laboratory analysis, and he is given IV clindamycin. A nurse marks the edges of the redness after consent from his mother. The resident thinks that the patient might have Ludwig angina.

Treatment

The patient is hospitalized because the cellulitis appears to be advancing rapidly. Intravenous antibiotics are continued.

Keep in Mind

Ludwig angina is an infection of the floor of the mouth usually originating from a dental infection. The tongue will frequently appear elevated. There is dysphagia and progressive airway obstruction. The word angina means strangling, which is why chest pain caused by myocardial ischemia is known as angina pectoris. Ludwig angina refers to the strangling sensation experienced by patients as the airway obstruction worsens.

This patient does not have Ludwig angina. His mouth appears normal, and there are no obvious dental caries. This appears to be a case of cellulitis of the neck. Cellulitis is usually caused by group A streptococci (GAS) or *Streptococcus aureus*. The cellulitis due to GAS usually encompasses a large area with a magenta hue referred to as an erythroderma. The cellulitis is generally flat and indurated, and the edges are often palpably raised slightly. Cellulitis due to *S aureus* is more limited and generally surrounds an abscess. The extent of the cellulitis is more localized.

Group A streptococci are sensitive to penicillin. Synergistic therapy with an anti–cell wall antibiotic (eg, penicillin) in conjunction with an anti-ribosomal antibiotic (eg, clindamycin) may be provided. Although GAS remains sensitive to penicillin, there is some clindamycin resistance. Inducible resistance to clindamycin has also been described with GAS; however, the frequency of resistance in the United States is currently low.

S aureus resistance to antistaphylococcal penicillins (eg, methicillin, oxacillin, nafcillin, cloxacillin) and cephalosporins has increased substantially in the past decade. Because most *S aureus* are now resistant (methicillin-resistant *S aureus* [MRSA]), treating suspected *S aureus* cellulitis infections with cephalosporins or antistaphylococcal penicillins is unwise. Methicillin-resistant *S aureus* is still mostly sensitive to vancomycin (IV only), clindamycin (only community acquired MRSA), trimethoprim-sulfamethoxazole, tetracycline, quinolones, and linezolid. Tetracyclines and quinolones are currently not used much in children because of the potential for adverse effects. Linezolid is expensive and restricted by many insurance company drug formularies. Sulfonamides have a higher risk of Stevens-Johnson syndrome and can precipitate hemolytic reactions in patients with glucose-6-phosphate dehydrogenase deficiency.

Clindamycin sensitivity might be overestimated (ie, resistance is underestimated) because of the phenomenon of inducible resistance. This is referred to as MLS resistance because this phenomenon occurs with macrolides, lincosamides, and streptogramins. The D-test illustrates the phenomenon of inducible MLS resistance. Figure 58-2 shows 2 Petri plates. The upper plate shows a growth of *S aureus* that is resistant to erythromycin (E) but sensitive to clindamycin (C) with a large zone of inhibition. The lower plate shows a growth of *S aureus* that is resistant to erythromycin (E). Note that there is a large zone of inhibition to the right of the clindamycin disk, but on the left, the presence of erythromycin has induced resistance to clindamycin. Note the tiny colonies of growth on the left side of the clindamycin disk. Inducible MLS resistance yields a D-shaped zone of inhibition, hence the descriptive term *positive D-test*. There are more sophisticated ways to check for inducible resistance, but these plates illustrate the phenomenon well.

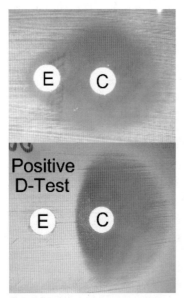

Figure 58-2

Recommended Reading

Fisher MC. Other anaerobic infections. In: Kliegman RM, Behrman RE, Jenson HB, Stanton BF, eds. *Nelson Textbook of Pediatrics.* 18th ed. Int ed. Philadelphia, PA: WB Saunders; 2007:1232–1235

Marr JK, Lim AT, Yamamoto LG. Erythromycin-induced resistance to clindamycin in *Staphylococcus aureus. Hawaii Med J.* 2005;64:6–8

Morelli JG. Cutaneous bacterial infections. In: Kliegman RM, Behrman RE, Jenson HB, Stanton BF, eds. *Nelson Textbook of Pediatrics.* 18th ed. Int ed. Philadelphia, PA: WB Saunders; 2007:2736–2745

Pascua LU. Cellulitis. In: Yamamoto LG, Inaba AS, Okamoto JK, Patronis ME, Yamashiroya VK, eds. *Case Based Pediatrics for Medical Students and Residents.* Honolulu, HI: University of Hawaii; 2004:183–186. Available at: http://www.hawaii.edu/medicine/pediatrics/pedtext. Accessed December 30, 2008

Chapter 59

Unilateral Neck Mass With Fever

Presentation

A 4-year-old boy arrives at your emergency department (ED) with a large right-sided neck mass. His temperature rose to 39°C 3 days previously. The next day, his physician prescribed amoxicillin for a left otitis media. Neck swelling and redness began 1 day before the current ED visit and increased in size despite antibiotic therapy. His family reports no ill contacts, no exposure to cats, no dental complaints, and no history of dental caries. His medical history is notable only for frequent courses of antibiotics for pharyngitis and otitis media.

At the time he presents, he is afebrile (37°C) and tachycardic (153 beats/ min) but normotensive (blood pressure 105/53 mm Hg). Although he is alert, he is irritable but consolable by his parents. An 6 × 6-cm firm mass arises from the right neck with erythema of the overlying skin. His left tympanic membrane is erythematous. He has no nuchal rigidity, but he keeps his head tilted to the left. His airway is patent and air entry is normal. He has no abdominal masses or adenopathy. No conjunctival, cutaneous, or extremity changes are present.

Discussion

Differential Diagnosis

- Lymphadenitis due to various infectious causes
  - Suppurative (eg, *Staphylococcus aureus,* group A streptococci, other oral and skin flora including anaerobes)
  - Viral
  - Less common bacterial pathogens (eg, *Corynebacterium diphtheriae,* mycobacteria, *Bartonella henselae* [cat-scratch disease])
  - Toxoplasma gondii
- Abscess
- Malignancy
- Branchial cleft cyst
- Kawasaki disease (KD), incomplete and early manifestation

Evaluation

Inflammatory indices include white blood cells 14,200/μL with 32% neutrophils and 35% band forms, C-reactive protein 32.6 mg/dL, and erythrocyte sedimentation rate 66 mm/h. Other hematologic values include hemoglobin 12.4 g/dL and platelets 332,000/μL. A contrast-enhanced computed tomography (CT) image of the neck, performed to evaluate for abscess and define the anatomy, reveals a solid 3 × 5 × 4-cm mass whose appearance suggests a cluster of reactive lymph nodes but that does not exclude neoplasm (figures 59-1 and 59-2). There is no evidence of airway compromise.

Treatment

In the ED, the patient's temperature increases to 38.7°C, and he receives acetaminophen orally and clindamycin intravenously (IV). Hypotension (blood pressure 68/46 mm Hg) develops after the patient returns from having a CT scan performed under sedation, and this raises concern for sepsis. Initial stabilization consists of rapid saline bolus infusions and broadening of antibiotic coverage with ceftriaxone and vancomycin before admission to the pediatric intensive care unit for close monitoring and pressor support.

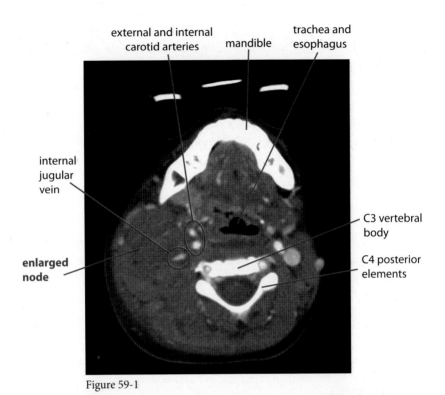

Figure 59-1

Figure 59-2

After admission for presumed bacterial adenitis and sepsis, hyperemia of the conjunctivae and lips, pedal edema, and urethral meatal inflammation become apparent. Additional studies reveal gamma glutamyl transferase 70 U/L (upper limit for age, 19 U/L), alanine aminotransferase 65 U/L, and pyuria (20–40 WBC per high-power field). His temperature peaks at 39.5°C, and he is diagnosed with KD. Fever and other clinical findings resolve after a single infusion of IV immunoglobulin (IVIG) 2 g/kg. Echocardiography reveals dilatation of the left anterior descending coronary artery, which resolves completely during convalescence.

Keep in Mind

Cervical adenopathy with or without fever is common in children. In most cases, clinical evaluation will uncover a benign or easily treated infectious cause without the use of diagnostic tests. Symptomatic therapy with or without empiric antibiotic coverage directed against staphylococci, streptococci, and possibly oral anaerobes is appropriate in the well-appearing child.

Kawasaki disease normally manifests as a constellation of fever and a combination of rash, conjunctival injection, cervical adenopathy, and mucous membrane and extremity changes. Cervical adenopathy is the least common of the principal criteria, appearing in approximately 50% of cases of KD. However, on occasion, KD will manifest initially with only fever and isolated adenopathy. In the absence of a specific diagnostic test, the diagnosis of KD will not be apparent until the clinical picture has evolved or an echocardiogram demonstrates characteristic changes of the coronary arteries. Although ultrasound is seldom performed in the evaluation of KD, it will demonstrate that a single palpable cervical mass consists of multiple nodes resembling a cluster of grapes.

Hypotension in acute KD is an increasingly recognized phenomenon and appears unrelated to myocarditis, myocardial ischemia, or IVIG infusion. Patients who present with a KD shock syndrome are more likely to have laboratory evidence of severe inflammation, thrombocytopenia, coronary artery abnormalities, and resistance to IVIG. They occasionally are admitted with competing diagnoses that may delay the definitive diagnosis and treatment for KD.

Because the differential diagnosis of a cervical mass includes other serious entities besides viral and bacterial disease, close outpatient monitoring of children with febrile cervical adenitis, along with strict instructions and precautions, is warranted until the illness resolves.

Recommended Reading

April MM, Burns JC, Newburger JW, Healy GB. Kawasaki disease and cervical adenopathy. *Arch Otolaryngol Head Neck Surg.* 1989;115: 512–514

Dominguez SR, Friedman K, Seewald R, Anderson MS, Willis L, Glodé MP. Kawasaki disease in a pediatric intensive care unit: a case-control study. *Pediatrics.* 2008;122:e786–e790

Kanegaye JT, Wilder MS, Molkara D, et al. Recognition of a Kawasaki disease shock syndrome. *Pediatrics.* 2009;123:e783–e789

Tashiro N, Matsubara T, Uchida M, Katayama K, Ichiyama T, Furukawa S. Ultrasonographic evaluation of cervical lymph nodes in Kawasaki disease. *Pediatrics.* 2002;109:e77

Waggoner-Fountain LA, Hayden GF, Hendley JO. Kawasaki syndrome masquerading as bacterial lymphadenitis. *Clin Pediatr (Phila).* 1995;34:185–189

Chapter 60

Neck Mass

Presentation

A 14-year-old boy is brought to the emergency department (ED) because his parents just noticed a large lump in his neck (Figure 60-1). He has no dysphagia, fever, cough, vomiting, or diarrhea. The teen indicates that he noticed this several months ago, but he thought it was his Adam's apple getting bigger. The ED physician asks about thyroid symptoms, to which the patient responds that he is an active boy who participates in sports. He doesn't have difficulty sleeping. He sweats a lot, but no more than usual, given his residence in Hawaii.

Past medical, social, and family histories are not contributory.

Examination reveals the following vital signs: oral temperature 37°C, pulse 90 beats/min, respiration 20 breaths/min, blood pressure 120/70 mm Hg, and oxygen saturation 99% in room air. He is small for his age, with a slender build. He is alert and cooperative. His examination is unremarkable with the exception of an enlarged, nontender thyroid. The enlarged thyroid is homogeneously firm. No nodules are palpable. His eyes appear normal (no exophthalmos).

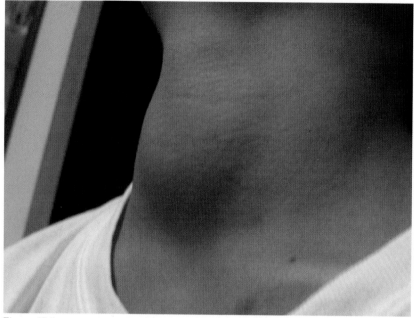

Figure 60-1

Discussion

Differential Diagnosis

- Mild hypertension
- Hyperthyroidism
- Thyroiditis
- Graves disease

Evaluation

Because the patient is clinically stable, his primary care physician is notified and a follow-up visit for the next day is arranged. Blood samples for thyroid studies are drawn in the ED. His parents are instructed to check on these test results tomorrow when they see their primary care physician.

His thyroid results the next day show a free T4 level of 3.9 ng/dL (normal range, 0.9–1.6 ng/dL), and a thyroid-stimulating hormone (TSH) level of 0.1 μIU/mL (normal range, 0.4–4.0 μIU/mL). These results indicate the presence of hyperthyroidism probably due to thyroiditis or Graves disease.

Treatment

Severe acute hyperthyroid symptoms can be controlled with propranolol. This was not necessary in this case. Long-term management options initiated by an endocrinologist include antithyroid drugs such as propylthiouracil (PTU) and methimazole (Tapazole), or partial thyroid ablation therapy with radiation or surgery. Propylthiouracil and methimazole can result in severe drug or hypersensitivity reactions that include manifestations such as rash, leukopenia, glomerulonephritis, vasculitis, and hepatitis.

Keep in Mind

Graves disease is an autoimmune thyroid condition in which autoantibodies mimic TSH. These autoantibodies, known as long-acting thyroid stimulators, occupy the TSH sites on the thyroid gland, stimulating the thyroid gland to synthesize and release excess levels of thyroid hormones. Patients with Graves disease may also develop other autoimmune conditions.

Symptoms of hyperthyroidism include hyperactivity, irritability, altered mood, insomnia, poor school performance, heat intolerance, increased sweating, pruritus, palpitations, weight loss, increased stooling frequency, polyuria, polydipsia, weakness, oligomenorrhea, or amenorrhea.

The initial phase of thyroiditis could also result in hyperthyroidism, which usually evolves to hypothyroidism. Specialized diagnostic testing can distinguish thyroiditis from Graves disease.

Recommended Reading

LaFranchi S. Disorders of the thyroid gland. In: Kliegman RM, Behrman RE, Jenson HB, Stanton BF, eds. *Nelson Textbook of Pediatrics.* 18th ed. Int ed. Philadelphia, PA: WB Saunders; 2007:2316–2348

Chapter 61

Neck Pain With C2-C3 Malalignment

Presentation

A 6-year-old girl is brought to the emergency department with a complaint of neck pain. Her parents describe her behavior as slightly different than normal. She doesn't want to walk around and she has not been moving her head much. The only history of trauma is having been thrown into a swimming pool about 32 hours ago. She did not complain of neck pain at the time, and she continued to play in the pool.

Examination reveals the following vital signs: temperature 37.0°C, pulse 120 beats/min, respiration 22 breaths/min, blood pressure 120/80 mm Hg, and oxygen saturation 100% on oxygen. She is crying and not very cooperative. Her head shows no signs of external trauma. Eyes, pupils, tympanic membranes, nose, and mouth examinations are normal. Her neck is difficult to examine, but she might have some tenderness over her posterior neck. Heart, lungs, and abdomen are normal. She moves all extremities well. Overall color and perfusion are good.

Discussion

Differential Diagnosis
- Mild cervical spine pain
- C2-C3 pseudosubluxation
- Traumatic cervical spine injury

Evaluation
The history of the traumatic injury suggests mild trauma. Your patient's only trauma was being thrown into a swimming pool 32 hours ago, at which time she did not complain of any pain and continued to swim and play in the pool. This sounds like mild trauma and a low-risk mechanism of injury.

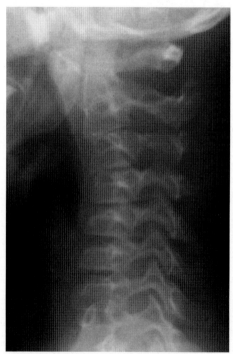

You order multiple radiographic views of her neck. The lateral view shows a malalignment of the vertebral bodies of C2-C3 (Figure 61-1). This finding most likely represents a pseudosubluxation as opposed to a true subluxation at her age.

Treatment
She is given acetaminophen, and a soft cervical collar is applied for comfort.

Figure 61-1

Keep in Mind

In children up to age 10 years, flexion and extension are greatest about C2 and C3. C2 may normally appear to be anterior relative to C3 by as much as 5 mm. This pseudosubluxation is increased if the radiograph is taken with the neck flexed. C2 simply flexes forward over C3. This finding may be present in as many as one third of all lateral cervical spine films in children.

The major true cervical spine injury that resembles pseudosubluxation is the so-called hangman fracture. There are several characteristics of a pseudosubluxation. All 4 of the following should be present: flexed positioning, mild trauma, mild pain, and posterior cervical line (described by Swischuk) within tolerances.

C2-C3 pseudosubluxation is only present when the neck is positioned in flexion. Ideally, the lateral cervical spine view should be taken with the patient's neck in extension (lordosis). However, many children are on spine boards and their large occiputs brings their heads and necks into relative flexion. In practice most of these radiographs are obtained in this position and this C2-C3 pseudosubluxation is a common radiographic finding in young children. If a C2-C3 malalignment is noted with the patient's neck in extension, this is more likely to be a true subluxation or fracture rather than a pseudosubluxation.

The degree of pain should be mild in a pseudosubluxation. It would be difficult to rule out a significant cervical spine injury based on plain film radiographs if the patient is complaining of severe pain. Such patients should be assessed by computed tomography or a magnetic resonance imaging scan of the cervical spine to more accurately establish whether a significant cervical spine injury is present.

The Swischuk line, or posterior cervical line, first described in 1977, is drawn from the posterior arch of C1 to the posterior arch of C3. The anterior cortex of the posterior arch of C2 should be within 1 mm of this line. In a true subluxation of C2, the arch of C2 would also be displaced anteriorly. The Swischuk line is drawn in the radiograph of the original patient (Figure 61-2). The longer line is the Swischuk line and the shorter line is the posterior arch of C2, which is within 1 mm of the Swischuk line.

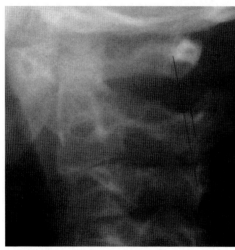

Figure 61-2

Figure 61-3 shows radiographs from another patient with C2-C3 malalignment. The neck is flexed. In this case, the Swischuk line (b) is perfectly intact; the posterior arches—C1, C2, and C3—line up. Similarly, in Figure 61-4, which shows radiographs from another patient with C2-C3 malalignment with a flexed neck, the arch of C1 is clearly visible. Again, the Swischuk line is perfectly intact (b).

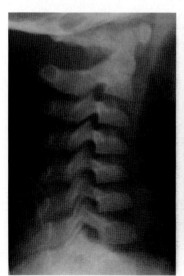

Figure 61-3a

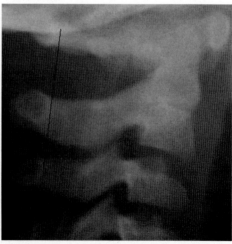

Figure 61-3b

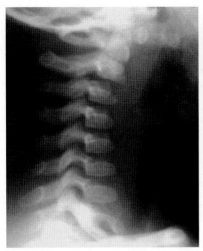

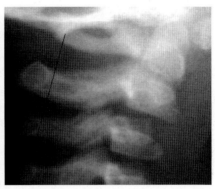

Figure 61-4b

Figure 61-4a

The Swischuk line should not be trusted in isolation to confirm a pseudo-subluxation. All 4 criteria should ideally be present. The radiographs in Figure 61-5 are of a child who was ejected from a car in a collision. Figure 61-5a shows C2-C3 malalignment. In Figure 61-5b, the Swischuk line is intact, but the white arrow points to a hangman fracture of the pedicle of C2. This fracture is produced when forces accelerate the head forward relative to a stationary neck, or when the neck is pulled backward relative to a stationary head.

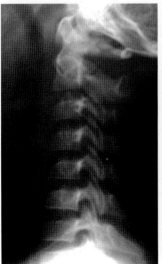

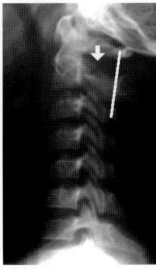

Figure 61-5a

Figure 61-5b

Recommended Reading

Lin TC, Yamamoto LG. Cervical spine radiographs. In: Yamamoto LG, Inaba AS, DiMauro R, eds. *Radiology Cases in Pediatric Emergency Medicine*. Vol 5, case 2. October 1996. Available at: http://www.hawaii.edu/medicine/pediatrics/pemxray/v5c02.html. Accessed December 31, 2008

Swischuk LE. Anterior displacement of C2 in children: physiologic or pathologic? A helpful differentiating line. *Radiology*. 1977;122:759–763

Yamamoto LG. Cervical spine malalignment—true or pseudo subluxation? In: Yamamoto LG, Inaba AS, DiMauro R, eds. *Radiology Cases in Pediatric Emergency Medicine*. Vol 1, case 5. November 1994. Available at: http://www.hawaii.edu/medicine/pediatrics/pemxray/v1c05.html. Accessed December 31, 2008

Yee LL. The hangman's fracture. In: Yamamoto LG, Inaba AS, DiMauro R, eds. *Radiology Cases in Pediatric Emergency Medicine*. Vol 5, case 3. October 1996. Available at: http://www.hawaii.edu/medicine/pediatrics/pemxray/v5c03.html. Accessed December 31, 2008

Chapter 62

Eye Pain

Presentation

A 14-year-old boy woke up after an afternoon nap complaining of bilateral eye burning. His mother put some over-the-counter eyedrops in his eyes. He was told to rest for a few hours, but he continued to complain that the pain worsened. He refused to open his eyes at all. His father thinks that something might have gotten in his eyes while he was watching his father do some home welding that afternoon, but the boy doesn't remember anything flying into his eyes. He went swimming in the community pool for about half an hour right after this.

Past medical history is negative.

Examination reveals the following vital signs: oral temperature 37.2°C, pulse 90 beats/min, respiration 24 breaths/min, and blood pressure 120/85 mm Hg. He is alert, but he refuses to open his eyes. Heart, lung, and abdominal examinations are negative. After some encouragement, he opens his eyes with some reservation. Intense bilateral conjunctival injection is noted. It is not possible to examine his fundi.

Discussion

Differential Diagnosis
- Burns to the eyes due to exposure to ultraviolet light
- Acute glaucoma
- Hyphema
- Corneal trauma

Evaluation
After oral analgesic and topical tetracaine eyedrops, fluorescein dye is instilled into both eyes. An examination under an ultraviolet light shows no corneal abrasions.

Treatment
The patient complained that the tetracaine drops burned a lot, and it did not alleviate his pain much. The patient is diagnosed as having ultraviolet light exposure burns. The patient's nonresponse to topical tetracaine suggests that the cause of the pain might be in the retina. This patient was provided with an oral narcotic analgesic (after telephone consultation with an ophthalmologist) and referred to an ophthalmologist for follow-up.

Keep in Mind
A welder's shield is worn to protect the eyes during welding. Physical particles can spray from the welding site. The welder's shield uses an ultraviolet light filter to prevent ultraviolet light exposure. Welding is achieved by variations of passing a high-voltage electrical arc creating heat or by burning a gas to achieve a high-temperature flame. These varying heat sources are combined with various types of metals to achieve welding conditions of different types. The bright glow of the welder's heat source on the metal emits intense visible light, but it also emits intense invisible light in the ultraviolet range. The ultraviolet eye shield filters this radiation, protecting the welder's eyes. Each welding type produces a different wavelength of ultraviolet radiation, so each welding type requires a different type of filter shield. Some of these filters are so thick that it appears completely black until the welding torch is turned on.

Similarly, a sunburn initially feels warm and comfortable, but several hours after the sun exposure, it becomes painful and red. The eye burns from ultraviolet exposure are similar. Note that in this case, while the boy observed the welding, he experienced no discomfort until several hours later. This condition is known as arc eye, which is an ultraviolet radiation exposure burn to the cornea and lens resulting in keratoconjunctivitis. Most of these cases are intensely painful but will resolve with time and do not result in a permanent threat to vision. However, some of these patients experience retinal burns as well, which are more serious.

A similar phenomenon, known as snow blindness, occurs while skiing at high altitudes. The high altitude permits more ultraviolet radiation and the white snow permits greater reflection of near-ultraviolet radiation. Simple ultraviolet eye protection is preventive.

Ultraviolet light exposure in tanning facilities also places clients at risk for ultraviolet eye injuries. Although the eyes are supposed to be covered and protected during ultraviolet light exposure, this protection results in so-called raccoon eyes, which are not aesthetically attractive. Thus, eye protection is often not used by tanning facility clients.

Topical ophthalmic anesthetics should eliminate discomfort coming from the external structures (cornea and conjunctiva). Tetracaine is commonly used, but it burns when initially instilled. Proparacaine is better because it is almost painless when instilled and it results in almost instant topical anesthesia.

Recommended Reading

Brittain GP. Retinal burns caused by exposure to MIG-welding arcs: report of two cases. *Br J Ophthalmol.* 1988;72:570–575

Levin AV. Eye—red. In: Fleisher GR, Ludwig S, Henretig FM, Ruddy RM, Silverman BK, eds. *Textbook of Pediatric Emergency Medicine.* 5th ed. Philadelphia, PA: Lippincott Williams & Wilkins; 2006:267–271

Lubeck D, Greene JS. Corneal injuries. *Emerg Med Clin North Am.* 1988;6:73–94

Walters BL, Kelley TM. Commercial tanning facilities: a new source of eye injury. *Am J Emerg Med.* 1987;5:386–389

Chapter 63

Facial Swelling

Presentation

A 15-year-old boy complains of cough of 1 month's duration and recent onset of face, upper trunk, and upper extremity swelling. He has also developed skin changes that he describes as "bruises" on the chest. For the last week, he has awoken with facial and neck swelling that improve but do not resolve completely during the day. He denies respiratory distress or positional dyspnea. His urine output has been normal in volume and character. He reports fatigue and joint pain, especially at night. He denies fever, night sweats, or weight loss. His hands have also become swollen. He denies dysphagia, abdominal pain, vomiting, diarrhea, scrotal pain or swelling, or lower extremity swelling. His treatment has consisted of an antihistamine for presumed allergies.

Family history is positive for seizures, asthma, adult heart disease, and cancer. He is afebrile with normal vital signs, room air oxyhemoglobin saturation of 96%, and normal perfusion and air movement. There is mild symmetric periorbital swelling with facial fullness and flushing. His upper extremities are diffusely edematous, and collateral vessels are visible on his upper chest (figures 63-1 and 63-2). He has no neck masses or jugular venous distention. Lung examination reveals clear respirations with no retractions or stridor. He has no adenopathy, abdominal masses, hepatosplenomegaly, ascites, or scrotal swelling.

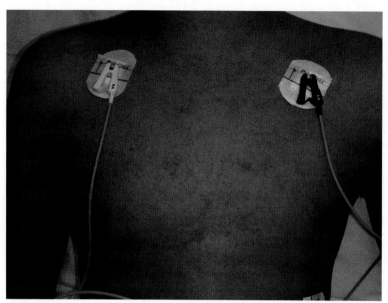

Figure 63-1

Figure 63-2

Discussion

Differential Diagnosis

- Infection (eg, tuberculosis, coccidioidomycosis and other fungal infections) or inflammatory condition (sarcoidosis)
- Neoplasm (eg, lymphoma, thymic tumor, germ cell tumor)
- Anatomic malformation such as lymphangioma
- Inhalational anthrax
- Edema due to renal or hepatic disease or congestive heart failure
- Vascular, such as hemorrhage associated with trauma

Evaluation

Hematologic evaluation includes white blood cell count 11,300/µL with normal differential and no blasts, hemoglobin 15.1 g/dL, and platelet count 185,000/µL. There is evidence of increased cell turnover (lactate dehydrogenase 2,450 U/L) but not of tumor lysis syndrome (potassium 4.6 mmol/L, calcium 9.3 mg/dL, phosphorus 4.2 mg/dL, uric acid 5.1 mg/dL). Chest radiography reveals mediastinal widening with retrosternal opacity, but no infiltrate (figures 63-3 and 63-4).

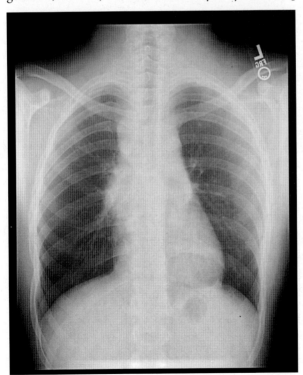

Figure 63-3

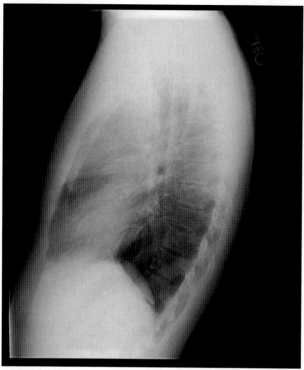

Figure 63-4

Treatment

You proceed promptly with stabilization, supportive measures, and evaluation of the patient's mass. On the basis of the mass and evidence of high cell turnover, your initial evaluation leads you to suspect malignancy. The primary concern is for potential airway and circulatory compromise. Because the patient is not experiencing respiratory distress and is able to lie supine without distress, computed tomography (CT) imaging is undertaken to define the mediastinal mass and the impingement on vascular and airway structures. Initial supportive care measures for suspected neoplasm include allopurinol and fluid hydration with alkalinization.

Computed tomography scan reveals a large (10 × 8 × 9 cm) anterior superior mediastinal mass (Figure 63-5) with obstruction of the superior vena cava (SVC) and extensive collateral flow (Figure 63-6). There is no hilar adenopathy. Because the mass does not impinge on the trachea or bronchi, critical care admission is not needed, and the patient is admitted to the oncology unit for further evaluation. Imaging of the abdomen and pelvis reveals no evidence of additional lymphadenopathy. Computed tomography–guided percutaneous needle biopsy is performed; analysis of the sample reveals a large B-cell lymphoma. Bone marrow biopsy and cerebrospinal fluid sampling are performed; neither reveals other evidence of malignancy. The oncology service initiates an aggressive chemotherapy regimen to rapidly reduce the tumor size.

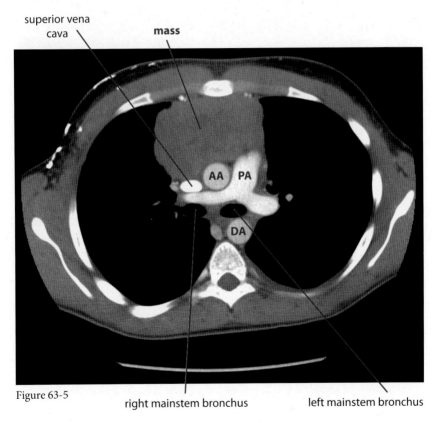

Figure 63-5

AA, ascending aorta; DA, descending aorta; PA, pulmonary artery.

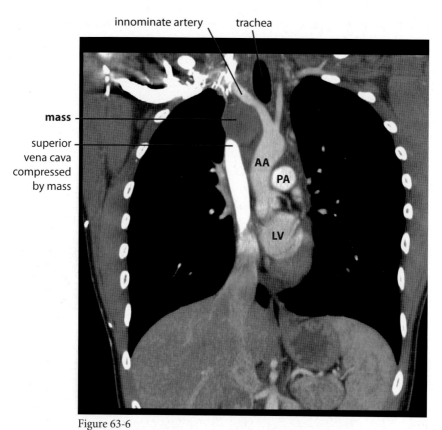

Figure 63-6

AA, ascending aorta; LV, left ventricle; PA, pulmonary artery.

Keep in Mind

The outpatient diagnosis of allergy is commonly made in the context of
facial swelling, but this may be misleading. Nephrotic syndrome may be
misdiagnosed initially as allergy. However, SVC syndrome is a rare but
more urgent and life-threatening condition to consider. Typical presenting
symptoms and signs of SVC syndrome include cough, dyspnea or ortho-
pnea, venous distention, and edema of the face and upper extremities.
The most common malignant cause of SVC syndrome in children is
non-Hodgkin lymphoma, whereas among adults, the most common
cause is bronchogenic carcinoma.

Superior mediastinal syndrome, or compression of the intrathoracic airway, is one of the most immediately life-threatening accompaniments of SVC syndrome. The emergency department (ED) clinician should avoid interventions that may further compromise the intrathoracic airway, such as sedation, induction of anesthesia, or neuromuscular blockade. Even the supine position required for CT imaging may be hard for the patient to tolerate. Initial therapy guided by tissue diagnosis is preferred, but empiric radiation and chemotherapy may be required if compromise of the airway or cardiac output precludes the induction of anesthesia.

Prompt multidisciplinary evaluation (oncology, critical care/anesthesia, and surgery) and management are warranted when SVC syndrome is suspected.

When a neoplasm with high cell turnover (leukemia, lymphoma) is strongly suspected, important tumor lysis precautions include hydration with potassium-free fluids, alkalinization, and agents to lower uric acid levels (ie, allopurinol, a xanthine oxidase inhibitor, or rasburicase, a recombinant form of urate oxidase). Although inpatient services familiar with pediatric oncology patients have well-developed protocols for the prevention and treatment of tumor lysis syndrome, initiation of precautions in the ED will expedite care, especially if the patient requires transport to a tertiary facility or if a delay will occur before inpatient orders are written. A practical initial solution for hydration and alkalinization is 5% dextrose in 0.25 normal saline with sodium bicarbonate 40 mEq/L infused at 1.5 times maintenance rate or greater to keep urine pH in the range of 7.0 to 7.5. The decision to administer allopurinol or rasburicase is best made in consultation with a pediatric oncologist; the latter agent, although very effective in high-risk cases, can falsely lower blood uric acid levels and carries a risk of anaphylaxis, methemoglobinemia, and hemolysis (in glucose-6-phosphate–deficient patients).

Recommended Reading

Rheingold SR, Lange BJ. Oncologic emergencies. In: Fleisher GR, Ludwig S, Henretig FM, Ruddy RM, Silverman BK, eds. *Textbook of Pediatric Emergency Medicine.* 5th ed. Philadelphia, PA: Lippincott Williams & Wilkins; 2006:1239–1274

Rheingold SR, Lange BJ. Oncologic emergencies. In: Pizza PA, Poplack DG. *Principles and Practice of Pediatric Oncology.* 5th ed. Philadelphia, PA: Lippincott Williams & Wilkins; 2006:1202–1230

Part 7

Extremity Presentations

Chapter 64

Femur Fracture and Suspected Child Abuse

Presentation

A 2-month-old boy is brought to the emergency department (ED) in the evening with a chief complaint of crying and fussiness. His mother reports that she was carrying him in a padded fabric infant carrier over the front of her body. His mother was also holding a lightweight cardboard gift box against his legs as she used this box to push the spring-loaded door open to enter their home. When she turned on the house lights as she opened the door, he let out a scream, then cried inconsolably for a while. Initially, his parents thought that the light awoke him from a nap, although his crying seemed excessive. Their next thought was that his arm had gotten caught in one of the straps of the infant carrier. Although he has calmed down since the incident, he still seems to be irritable and uncomfortable. He feeds well, but he is intermittently fussy. There is no history of fever, vomiting, or cold symptoms. Before this, he seemed to be fine. He passed 2 normal stools earlier in the day.

Past medical history is negative.

When you examine the boy, you record the following vital signs: tympanic temperature 36.9°C, pulse 110 beats/min, respiration 40 breaths/min, and oxygen saturation 100% in room air. He is alert and interactive, in no distress. He is not toxic appearing. He is not crying and does not appear to be irritable when bounced. During various aspects of the examination, he is crying intermittently, but this appears to be a normal reaction to an examiner. His anterior fontanelle is soft and flat. His head has no swelling or tenderness. His neck is supple. His heartbeat is regular without murmurs. His lungs are clear. His abdomen is soft and nontender; no hernias are present. His testes and penis are normal. His clavicles are nontender, as is his back. Hip range of motion is good. There is no consistent reaction when palpating his upper and lower extremities. His digits and penis are examined for hair tourniquets and none are found. Perfusion and color are good.

Discussion

Differential Diagnosis
- Colic
- Intussusception
- Appendicitis

Evaluation
The possibility of intussusception is discussed. The abdomen is reexamined. Crepitus is noted in his left lower extremity when it is reexamined. Although focal tenderness was not obvious to the examiner or to his parents earlier, moving his left leg now consistently elicits discomfort.

Radiographs of his left lower extremity are obtained, and they reveal an angulated oblique fracture of the femur (Figure 64-1). A high-risk set of circumstances for suspecting child abuse occurs when the documented

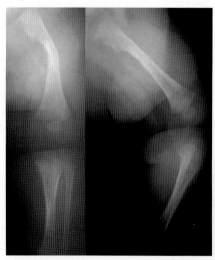
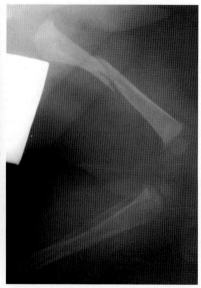

Figure 64-1

injury is not consistent with the history of the injury. You do not think that the history of this injury is consistent with these radiographic findings; because this is a femur fracture, there should be a history of substantial trauma, but history is lacking in this case.

The parents are confronted with the child's radiographs. They are asked if there is any other possible injury that they have neglected to tell the physician. They cannot recall any other possible trauma. His mother now believes that the door may have hit the box she was carrying at the time, and this box might have hit him in the leg. She is told that such an injury would require a force greater than this. She agrees and is similarly puzzled because she points out that the thin gift box should not have been hard enough to cause a fracture.

Because of the possibility of child abuse, other radiographs are obtained to look for older occult fractures. Radiographs of the patient's upper extremities are shown in Figure 64-2. No significant abnormalities are identified. Radiographs in child abuse cases will sometimes demonstrate healing fractures and periosteal elevation resulting from healing bony injuries.

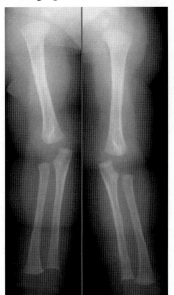

Figure 64-2

Treatment
The family is informed that this case needs to be reported to child protective services.

An orthopedic surgeon places the child in a hip spica cast. The ED physician notes that the history of the fracture does not account for the radiographic finding, but it is a highly unusual story. In most cases of child abuse, the history given will usually be that the child fell off the couch or bed, or his leg got caught in the crib railings. In this case, the history is that the infant's leg was compressed against a door and a thin cardboard gift box. These parents are intelligent, and they agree that they don't understand how this could possibly cause such a large fracture in such a big bone. If this were a case of child abuse, the perpetrator would not likely provide an implausible story. How can the risk of child abuse be further ascertained?

Child protective services arrive and interview the parents in the ED. The police officer and child protective service worker agree that this story is unusual and is not typical of child abuse, yet the radiographic findings are undeniable. The patient's primary care physician is called, and he adamantly states that this family is absolutely not capable of child abuse. He requests that the child be discharged from the ED, and he will see the patient tomorrow and maintain responsibility for follow-up.

Further history on this family is that there are several family members with frequent fractures. The infant's father has had 3 fractures, and he notes that the trauma that caused the fractures was not very severe. He also notes that his father (the infant's paternal grandfather) also had several fractures just from "horsing around." His mother has a history of scoliosis. Other relatives have a history of scoliosis and bowleggedness.

The patient is discharged from the ED after all parties—the orthopedic surgeon, primary care physician, child protective service worker, and police officer—agree. The next day, the radiologist comments that the bones are slightly demineralized and the skull views might be consistent with the presence of wormian bones. Genetic testing confirms the presence of osteogenesis imperfecta (OI).

Keep in Mind

In most instances, it is advisable to inform parents whenever a report to child protective services is made. This is because they may be very unhappy when they find out that such a report has been made. A less threatening way to inform parents that a report is about to be made is to approach them in a nonjudgmental and objective manner. Put the radiograph with the femur fracture on the view box or computer screen and while pointing to the fracture, inform them that there is a government law that requires us to report this type of injury to child protective services. While pointing to the fracture, say, "Whenever this type of injury occurs, it must be reported. Child protective services will be contacting you. Just tell them what happened." Parents perceive that it is the radiographic injury that is being reported, not them personally. Similarly, if a child comes in with multiple bruises and burns due to a history that is not plausible, parents should be informed that the government laws require that "this type of injury" (while pointing to the injury) must be reported to child protective services. Parents perceive that the injuries are being reported and not them personally. This is true in many ways because the actual perpetrator cannot usually be determined with certainty during the initial medical encounter. This approach is less judgmental and results in less of an adverse reaction.

Figure 64-3 is from a different patient who has a femur fracture. The large oblique portion of the fracture is obvious. However, the fracture extends all the way to the distal femur. Also note that this patient's upper extremity radiographs demonstrate an old fracture in the radius (Figure 64-4 [left]) and the other lower extremity shows extensive periosteal elevation over the entire tibia (Figure 64-4 [right]).

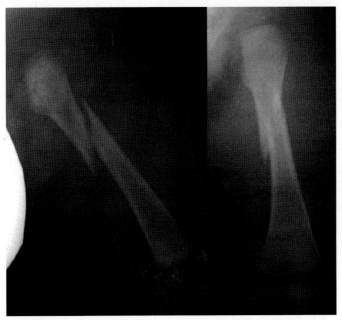

Figure 64-3

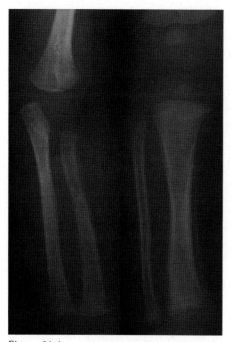

Figure 64-4

There are several different types of OI that will not be discussed here. The blue sclerae finding is classic, but it is only present in some patients, and this finding might be transient. As a general principle, the severe type of OI that is incompatible with life beyond childhood is inherited in an autosomal-recessive pattern. Some are new mutations. Lethal genetic conditions are autosomal-recessive, X-linked recessive, or new mutations because this is the only way that the allele can survive in the gene pool. If a lethal-condition allele was dominant, it would not survive to the next generation.

Figure 64-5 is a chest radiograph from a 3-month-old with the severe type of OI that demonstrates severe osteopenia and multiple healing rib fractures (the bulbous findings on the ribs) (Figure 64-6). This patient's upper extremities (Figure 64-7) demonstrate severe osteopenia and crumpled bones, as do the lower extremities (Figure 64-8).

In the more occult type of OI that often manifests as frequent fractures, the osteopenia is not as obvious. Except for new mutations, this type is more often inherited in an autosomal-dominant pattern. Thus, there is usually a family history of frequent fractures in one of the parents.

For patients with fractures, asking about previous fractures could be useful in identifying patients with OI. In patients with several previous fractures, a follow-up question of whether any of the parents or siblings had frequent fractures could be useful. Genetic testing is required for patients suspected of having OI.

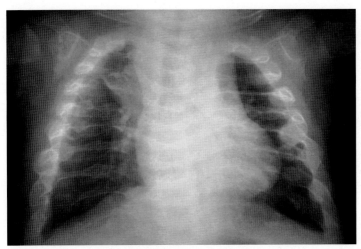

Figure 64-5

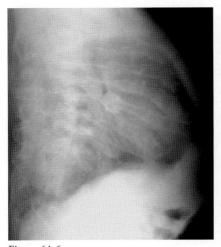

Figure 64-6

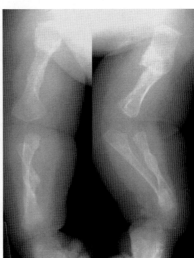

Figure 64-7

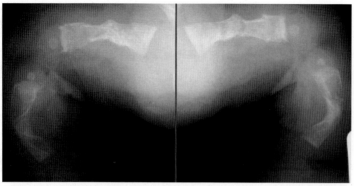

Figure 64-8

Fractures in OI patients are often mistaken for child abuse. The diagnosis of the occult forms of OI is not easy to establish in the ED; however, a positive family history might help to identify some patients with OI.

Recommended Reading

Boychuk RB. Sudden thigh swelling in a 6-week-old infant. In: Yamamoto LG, Inaba AS, DiMauro R, eds. *Radiology Cases in Pediatric Emergency Medicine.* Vol 2, case 17. March 1995. Available at: http://www.hawaii.edu/medicine/pediatrics/pemxray/v2c17.html. Accessed December 31, 2008

Yamamoto LG. Fussiness following minor trauma in an infant. In: Yamamoto LG, Inaba AS, DiMauro R, eds. *Radiology Cases in Pediatric Emergency Medicine.* Vol 6, case 2. July 1999. Available at: http://www.hawaii.edu/medicine/pediatrics/pemxray/v6c02.html. Accessed December 31, 2008

Yamamoto LG. Vomiting and coughing in a 3-month-old with weak bones. In: Yamamoto LG, Inaba AS, DiMauro R, eds. *Radiology Cases in Pediatric Emergency Medicine.* Vol 6, case 3. July 1999. Available at: http://www.hawaii.edu/medicine/pediatrics/pemxray/v6c03.html. Accessed December 31, 2008

Chapter 65

Severe Joint Pain

Presentation

A 12-year-old boy is brought to the emergency department because of a 7-hour complaint of severe ankle pain and fever. He is unable to walk. There is no obvious swelling and no history of trauma.

Past medical history based on recall is negative.

Your examination reveals the following vital signs: oral temperature 38.5°C, pulse 100 beats/min, respiration 35 breaths/min, blood pressure 110/80 mm Hg, and weight in the 25th percentile. He is alert and still, occasionally crying from pain. Examination of head, eyes, ears, nose, and throat is normal. The neck is supple. Heartbeat is regular with no murmur. Lungs are clear. The abdomen is soft and nontender. The child is neurologically intact. Very slight swelling is visible about the right ankle with no redness. His ankle is extremely tender when touched, and range of motion elicits severe pain. His foot is also tender. He is unable to walk or bear weight.

Discussion

Differential Diagnosis
- Acute rheumatic fever (ARF)
- Early septic arthritis
- Occult trauma
- Occult fracture
- Juvenile rheumatoid arthritis
- Toxic synovitis

Evaluation
Complete blood count reveals the following: white blood cells 19,100/μL, 75% segmented neutrophils, 15% lymphocytes, 10% monocytes, hemoglobin 12 g/dL, hematocrit 36%, and platelet count 420,000/μL.

Laboratory evaluation reveals an erythrocyte sedimentation rate of 100 mm/hr and a C-reactive protein value of 20 mg/dL. Chest radiograph and electrocardiogram are normal. Echocardiogram reveals mild mitral insufficiency.

The patient is diagnosed with presumptive ARF.

Treatment
The patient is hospitalized and treated with ibuprofen and penicillin. On arrival on the ward, he indicates that his left shoulder is also painful. By the next day, his ankle pain has resolved and he is able to walk. His shoulder pain resolves as well. Streptococcal serology is highly positive.

Keep in Mind
Acute rheumatic fever is an autoimmune subacute complication of untreated group A streptococcal infections. The incidence of ARF has continued to decline for reasons that are not fully understood.

Acute rheumatic fever is diagnosed by the Jones criteria. Establishing the diagnosis requires evidence of a preceding streptococcal infection via serology or culture plus either 1 major plus 2 minor criteria, or 2 major criteria. Major criteria include carditis, migratory polyarthritis, erythema marginatum, Sydenham chorea, or subcutaneous nodules. Minor criteria include fever, arthralgia, high acute-phase reactants, leukocytosis, and first-degree atrioventricular block (prolonged P–R interval).

In children with classic ARF, of the major Jones criteria, migratory polyarthritis is the most common. The patient will generally complain of severe joint pain in one joint. Similar findings will develop in another joint as migration occurs, as in this patient. Arthralgia is a subjective sensation of joint discomfort, whereas arthritis demonstrates objective evidence of joint inflammation as manifested by any of the following: visible swelling, redness, heat, diminished range of motion, painful range of motion, or direct joint tenderness. Some of these are more applicable to some joints than others. For example, it is not possible to visualize swelling about the hip joint, but palpation and range of motion are assessable. The carpal and tarsal joints of the hands and feet, respectively, cannot be put through range of motion, but swelling, redness, or palpable tenderness can be assessed.

Carditis is the next most common major Jones criterion. Carditis is most classically manifested as valvulitis of the mitral or aortic valves. Acute valvulitis manifests as valvular insufficiency. Mitral insufficiency is classically auscultated as a holosystolic murmur at the apex radiating into the axilla. Aortic insufficiency is classically auscultated as a soft diastolic murmur at the base. Echocardiography can demonstrate mild degrees of valvular regurgitation that are not apparent clinically; however, some of these are not necessarily indicative of clinically significant carditis or valvulitis. As the inflammatory process subsides, the valvular inflammation potentially scars, resulting in the valvular stenosis known as rheumatic heart disease (as opposed to ARF). Carditis can less commonly manifest as pericarditis, myocarditis, or advanced-degree (second- or third-degree) atrioventricular block (not first-degree arterioventricular block because this is a minor Jones criterion); however, because these more commonly result from viral or postviral processes other than ARF, it is more difficult to attribute these manifestations of carditis to ARF.

Severe joint tenderness with a rapid and dramatic response to nonsteroidal antiinflammatory drugs is classic for ARF.

Although the overall incidence of ARF has been reported to be low, recent reports in the literature demonstrate high incidence reporting in Hawaii and western Pennsylvania.

Recommended Reading

American Heart Association, Council of Cardiovascular Disease in the Young, Special Writing Group of the Committee on Rheumatic Fever, Endocarditis, and Kawasaki Disease. Guidelines for the diagnosis of rheumatic fever. Jones Criteria, 1992. *JAMA.* 1992;268:2069–2073

Erdem G, Mizumoto C, Esaki D, et al. Group A streptococcal isolates temporally associated with acute rheumatic fever in Hawaii: differences from the continental United States. *Clin Infect Dis.* 2007;45:e20–e24

Ferrieri P, for the Jones Criteria Working Group. Proceedings of the Jones Criteria Workshop (AHA Scientific Statement). *Circulation.* 2002;106:2521–2523

Martin JM, Barbadora KA. Continued high caseload of rheumatic fever in western Pennsylvania: possible rheumatogenic emm types of *Streptococcus pyogenes. J Pediatr.* 2006;149:58–63

Reddy DV, Chun LT, Yamamoto LG. Acute rheumatic fever with advanced degree AV block. *Clin Pediatr.* 1989;28:326–328

Chapter 66

Limping After a Fall

Presentation

A 20-month-old girl is brought to the emergency department (ED) at about 9:00 pm by her parents with a complaint that she will not stand on her right leg since earlier this evening. Parents are unsure of any trauma, but recently she has been falling when trying to run. The pattern of her crying makes her parents think that the pain originates from her knee. There is no history of fever or prodromal symptoms, and there is no history of previous injuries. Her parents report that she is able to walk, but with a limp. Her past medical history is significant only for wheezing.

Your examination reveals the following vital signs: temperature 37°C, pulse 127 beats/min, respiration 24 breaths/min, blood pressure 113/79 mm Hg, and weight 12.8 kg. She is apprehensive when people approach but is alert and otherwise comfortable, in no acute distress. Examination of head, eyes, ears, nose, and throat is negative for any signs of external trauma or other abnormalities. Her neck is supple. Her heartbeat is regular without murmurs. Her lungs are clear. Her abdomen is soft, flat, and nontender, with normoactive bowel sounds and no masses. Color and perfusion are good. She has good range of motion of all joints with no deformities or effusions. You note no erythema, warmth, or abrasions. No definite area of tenderness can be determined at examination. When you observe her gait, you notice that she will not fully bear weight on the right leg. She takes a few steps, walking very slowly with a limp.

Discussion

Differential Diagnosis

- Fracture
- Contusion

Evaluation

A radiograph of her entire right lower extremity is obtained (Figure 66-1; only the tibia-fibula portion is shown here). This is read as normal. She is instructed to follow up with her primary care physician tomorrow.

The next morning, the hospital radiologist reviewing the radiograph shown in Figure 66-1 calls the ED to notify the ED physician that the patient might have a small fracture in the distal tibia. Additional radiographic views are recommended.

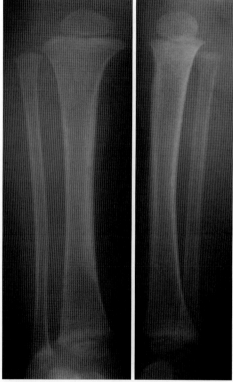

The patient is called, and on returning to the radiography department, she is now walking normally. Additional views of her tibia are obtained (Figure 66-2).

The original radiograph is shown in Figure 66-3 at left; the repeat radiograph is on the right. The same radiographs are shown in Figure 66-4 with the white arrow pointing to a nondisplaced oblique fracture of the distal third of the right tibia. It is a thin lucency that is difficult to see. The black arrow with the white outline points to a vascular groove.

Figure 66-1

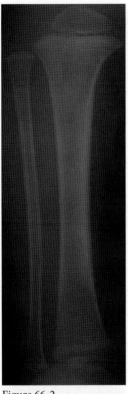

Figure 66-2

Treatment

A posterior splint is placed on the patient's lower leg, and she is referred to orthopedics. Given the oblique nature of this fracture, could this injury be due to child abuse?

Keep in Mind

Fractures found in small children with a history of very mild or no trauma must alert the clinician to possible nonaccidental injury. However, the diagnosis of child abuse can bring about serious consequences for the suspected perpetrator, family, and child. Thus, clinicians must be careful when evaluating cases of possible child abuse and not arrive at a conclusion too quickly. Various conditions can be mistaken for abuse, so an accurate history must be obtained, a thorough physical examination performed, and the necessary studies conducted to arrive at the correct conclusion.

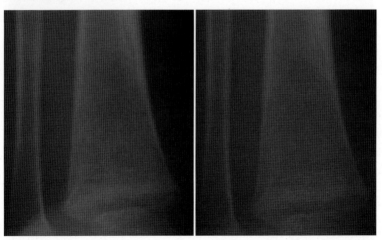

Figure 66-3

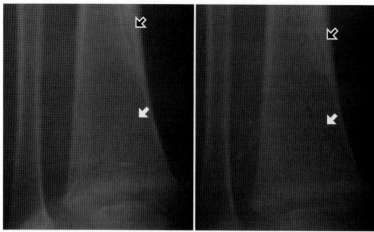

Figure 66-4

In our patient, this fracture represents a typical toddler's fracture, described as a subtle, nondisplaced oblique fracture of the distal tibia in children aged 9 months to 3 years. The child usually experiences an acute onset of limp or refusal to bear weight on one leg. Toddlers are still learning to walk, and they often attempt to run as well. They might twist their feet during one of their many falls.

Radiographic findings are frequently subtle, as in our case. Because the plane of the fracture is thin, the fracture will not be visible radiographically unless it is nearly parallel to the x-ray beam. If the view is slightly oblique, the fracture will be difficult to see. There is a high likelihood of having a toddler's fracture in a limping toddler, even if the initial radiographs are negative. Splinting all such patients is prudent, although this kind of fracture is stable.

Osteomyelitis, septic arthritis, and hip problems are always possibilities in a limping child; thus, identification of the toddler's fracture will confirm the fracture as the cause of the limping and will reduce or eliminate the need to evaluate the child further.

The toddler's fracture is a small distal tibia fracture. Such fractures are not associated with other known instances of child abuse. However, midshaft tibia fractures have been associated with child abuse. Large (as opposed to small) distal tibia fractures can also be accidental. This phenomenon is more common in 2- to 6-year-old children, as opposed to the smaller distal tibia classic toddler's fracture occurring in 9-month-old to 3-year-old children. This makes distinguishing accidents from child abuse more difficult. Following these classic age groupings can be helpful. For example, a large spiral fracture of the distal tibia in an infant is not likely to be an accidental toddler's fracture.

Accidental fractures in general are more likely to be isolated (except in major multiple trauma). Patients will seek care promptly after injury with a history that fits the fracture pattern. On the other hand, fractures in a child resulting from child abuse may be multiple and at various stages of healing. Inflicted skeletal trauma may involve any part of the skeleton. The presentation is often delayed with an unclear history or a minor injury that does not fit the fracture pattern. For example, a femur fracture in a preambulatory child should raise the suspicion of nonaccidental trauma.

It is not always easy to distinguish accidental from inflicted trauma. A classic toddler's fracture is unlikely to be caused by child abuse. Large fractures in nonambulatory infants are suspicious for child abuse. When child abuse is suspected or it is unclear, the law requires that child protective services be notified.

Recommended Reading
Alexander JE, Fizrandolph RL, McConnel JR. The limping child. *Curr Probl Diagn Radiol.* 1987;16:231–270

Dunbar JS, Owen HF, Nograday MM, et al. Obscure tibial fracture of infants—the toddler's fracture. *J Can Assoc Radiol.* 1964;15:136–144

Mellick LB, Reesor K. Spiral tibial fractures of children: a commonly accidental spiral long bone fracture. *Am J Emerg Med.* 1990;8:234–237

Santhany MD. The toddler's fracture: accident or child abuse? In: Yamamoto LG, Inaba AS, DiMauro R, eds. *Radiology Cases in Pediatric Emergency Medicine.* Vol 4, case 18. January 1996. Available at: http://www.hawaii.edu/medicine/pediatrics/pemxray/v4c18.html. Accessed December 31, 2008

Tenenbein M, Reed MH, Black GB. The toddler's fracture revisited. *Am J Emerg Med.* 1990;8:208–211

Chapter 67

Heel Pain

Presentation

A 14-year-old boy presents with a complaint of pain over the back of both his heels. He is brought in by his father after football practice because he has been having these pains for 2 weeks now. He says that it becomes sore toward the end of practice, and it has been especially bothersome today. He has had several ankle sprains in the past, but this feels different. The team trainer told him that he needs a doctor's note if he is to continue playing.

Past medical history is negative except for 3 ankle sprains.

Examination reveals the following vital signs: oral temperature 37.1°C, pulse 70 beats/min, respiration 18 breaths/min, and blood pressure 120/80 mm Hg. He is alert and active. Examination of his feet reveals moderate tenderness when compressing the back of his heels. He walks well and is able to jump up and down. There are no visible bruising, wounds, or deformity. There are no other areas of tenderness. His ankles have normal range of motion without discomfort.

Discussion

Differential Diagnosis

- Sever disease
- Occult bone condition
- Occult fracture

Evaluation

Radiographs of the patient's feet are obtained. One side is shown in Figure 67-1. The main point of interest in this case is the heel at the Achilles tendon insertion. The oblique view shows crescent-shaped lucencies over the posterior calcaneus in the area of concern (Figure 67-2). These lucencies represent the growth plate viewed obliquely. The lateral view shows the physis in a truly lateral view. These radiographs of the foot are normal.

You diagnose the patient as having Sever disease.

Treatment

The patient is instructed to rest when the pain occurs and to reduce stress on the tendon insertion site.

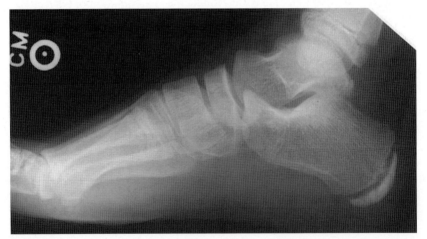

Figure 67-1

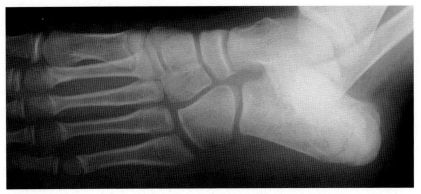

Figure 67-2

Keep in Mind

The most common cause of heel pain in adolescents is calcaneal apophysitis, or Sever disease. Radiographs of the heel are usually considered to be normal, as they were in this patient.

An apophysis is a growth plate that does not contribute to the length of the bone. The Achilles tendon inserts in the calcaneal apophysis. The growth plate is apparent in the radiograph in Figure 67-1. The growth plate is weak and subject to microinjury if there is excessive force placed on it. Under high-performance athletic stress, extreme tension is applied by the calf muscles via the Achilles tendon. Microinjury (microseparation) occurs at the apophysis, resulting in pain, a condition known as Sever disease.

A similar condition that is more commonly described is Osgood-Schlatter disease, in which the patellar tendon stresses the tibial tuberosity apophysis. Under high-performance athletic stress, the quadriceps pull on the patella, patella tendon, and patella tendon insertion into the tibial tuberosity apophysis. Microinjury (microseparation) occurs at the apophysis, resulting in pain. The pain is reproduced when the tibial tuberosity is compressed. The tibial tuberosity is often prominent and sometimes visibly inflamed.

Maximum pull on the patellar tendon and its insertion into the tibial tuberosity occur with maximal quadriceps contraction. Jumping is the most common major stress resulting in Osgood-Schlatter disease. Volleyball players and basketball players frequently jump forcefully during practice and games.

Kicking a soccer ball results in forceful quadriceps contraction, but a soccer ball is much lighter than the body, which is why Osgood-Schlatter is more common among volleyball and basketball players than soccer players. Weight lifters also forcefully extend the knees, which requires forceful quadriceps contraction and maximal pulling stress on the tibial tendon insertion. However, this is not as repetitive as in volleyball and basketball.

In Sever disease, maximum pull on the Achilles tendon occurs with forceful plantar flexion of the foot. The force is maximal in athletes who wear cleats on their shoes. The cleats provide the athlete with additional grip in the ground, permitting the gastrocnemius to apply maximal stress on the Achilles tendon. Baseball players wearing metal cleats who are sprinting while running the bases apply enough force on the Achilles tendon insertion to cause Sever disease. Football players wearing cleats who are pushing hard against other players, such as the ball carrier (eg, halfback, fullback, tailback) and offensive linemen, place great stress on the Achilles tendon insertion, which places the athlete at risk for Sever disease. Examination of the heel typically reveals tenderness to compression of the medial and lateral sides of the calcaneal apophysis and decreased dorsiflexion of the ankle without any swelling or erythema. Findings are bilateral in about 60% of patients. Radiographs are generally not necessary.

Sever and Osgood-Schlatter diseases are overuse injuries that will resolve with time as the growth plates fuse. Before closure of the growth plate, players must apply less force (eg, rest) on the tendon insertion when pain occurs. Successful treatment for Sever disease includes foam heel pads to elevate the heel and reduce the stretch of the Achilles tendon. Physical therapy with gastrocnemius-soleus stretching and dorsiflexion strengthening has been useful as well. Discontinuing aggravating activities is probably the simplest treatment. Instructing patients to rest when the pain worsens allows them to continue in their sports without the need for orthopedic restrictions.

Although younger children have weaker tendon insertions, they are lighter (less of a force when they jump and push against other players), and they are not practicing and working out as hard as teen athletes, who are more serious about high-performance athletic competition.

Recommended Reading

Nakano EA. Sever's disease. In: Yamamoto LG, Inaba AS, DiMauro R, eds. *Radiology Cases in Pediatric Emergency Medicine.* Vol 1, case 20. November 1994. Available at: http://www.hawaii.edu/medicine/pediatrics/pemxray/v1c20.html. Accessed December 31, 2008

Chapter 68

Cold, Pulseless Limb

Presentation

A 5-day-old girl is brought to the emergency department with a cold left leg. Her mother noted during an early morning diaper change that her daughter's left foot was slightly more pale than her right. Several hours later, when she was dressing the baby, the left lower extremity was distinctly cool below the knee, with a bluish tinge and a deeper discoloration over the left great toe. There were no other abnormal symptoms such as fever, rhinorrhea, cough, respiratory distress, vomiting, diarrhea, feeding, altered mental status, or rash. The mother reports that pregnancy and delivery were uncomplicated, and there had been no umbilical vessel catheterization or needle punctures in the affected leg. After 2 days in the hospital, she was discharged after an unremarkable 2-day nursery stay. There is no family history of hypercoagulable state, thrombosis, or cerebrovascular accident.

The infant is afebrile and has normal vital signs. She is well perfused except in the left leg (Figure 68-1). She weighs 2.4 kg—substantially less than her birth weight of 2,850 g. She is awake, alert, and vigorous. Her heart rate and rhythm are regular, and there is no murmur. The abdomen is soft and without masses. The left leg is cool and dusky below the knee, with a hemorrhagic region on the lateral aspect of the left great toe (Figure 68-2). Femoral pulses are palpable but diminished on the left, with no pulses palpable distally on the left leg. Her skin has no rashes.

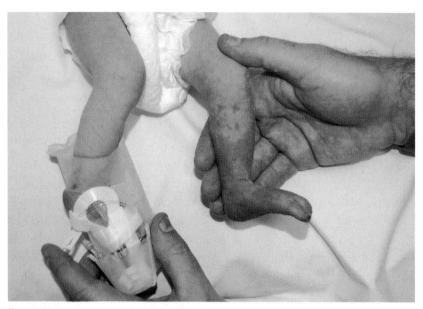

Figure 68-1

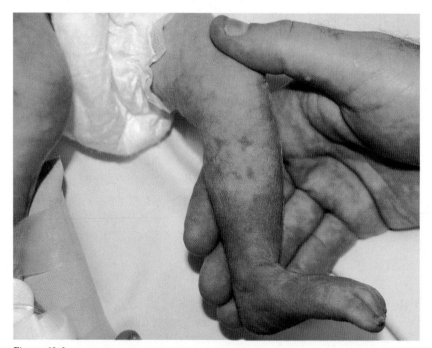

Figure 68-2

Discussion

Differential Diagnosis

- Hypercoagulable state
- Embolus
- Vasospasm
- Complication of vascular device or trauma
- Dehydration/shock
- Inflicted trauma

Evaluation

Isolated pallor or cold limb in an otherwise well-perfused pink infant make cardiovascular, pulmonary, or infectious causes unlikely. You use a hand-held Doppler device to confirm the absence of distal pulses.

You coordinate care with the neonatal intensive care unit (NICU) team and the radiology department. Ultrasonography demonstrates a noncompressible, echogenic left common femoral artery with no flow, consistent with thrombus formation.

Treatment

After admission to the NICU, angiography confirms occlusion of the left iliac and femoral arteries. She undergoes intraarterial infusion of tissue plasminogen activator with rapid improvement in perfusion (Figure 68-3). She receives fluid hydration for hypernatremic dehydration (sodium 161 mmol/L). Echocardiogram reveals no intracardiac shunts, thrombi, or vegetations. However, a large patent ductus arteriosus is identified and ligated.

Anticoagulation therapy is initiated with low-molecular-weight heparin and continued on an outpatient basis. Follow-up ultrasonography reveals restoration of flow in the arteries of the left leg with some residual resistance. A venous thrombosis panel reveals no evidence of hypercoagulability. Normal flow is present at a 2-month follow-up ultrasound examination.

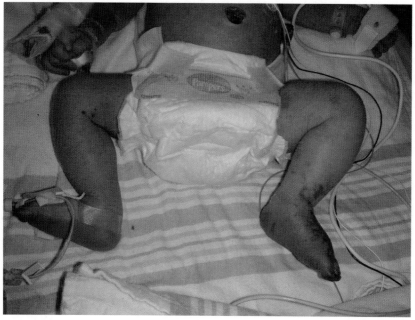

Figure 68-3

Keep in Mind

Thromboembolic events are uncommon in children, although premature neonates who have undergone umbilical vessel catheterization are at higher risk. Development of a thrombus depends on abnormalities of the vessel (catheter), flow (eg, polycythemia, dehydration, shock), or coagulation (prethrombotic disorders such as activated protein C resistance and deficiencies of protein C or S). Usually more than one risk factor is present. The single most common cause is a current or prior vascular catheter. Other important risk factors include asphyxia, sepsis, dehydration, maternal diabetes, and cardiac disease. Renal vein thrombosis is the most common noncatheter-related thrombotic complication.

When the obstruction is in the peripheral circulation, the clinical findings are usually highly suggestive of the diagnosis. Less-specific manifestations with deeper vessels include cardiovascular, neurologic, and respiratory symptoms and signs. Many thrombotic events probably go unrecognized if the patient has few symptoms. In this case, hypernatremic dehydration and the hemodynamic disturbance due to the patent ductus arteriosus are contributory.

Investigation of underlying thrombotic conditions is outside of the scope of emergency management. However, consultation with a hematologist early in the course of treatment may help guide the diagnostic evaluation, the results of which may be affected by therapy. Even in the absence of a known cause, ED priorities include recognition of a potentially limb- or life-threatening condition, support of vital function with attention to correction of underlying hemodynamic disturbances, and initiation of multidisciplinary management (ie, radiology, neonatology or critical care, hematology).

Recommended Reading

Blanchette V, Dror Y, Chan A. Hematology. In: MacDonald MG, Seshia MMK, Mullett MD, eds. *Avery's Neonatology: Pathophysiology and Management of the Newborn.* 6th ed. Philadelphia, PA: Lippincott Williams & Wilkins; 2005:1168–1234

Chalmers EA, Gibson BE. Hemostatic problems in the neonate. In: Lilleyman JS, Hann IM, Blanchette VS, eds. *Pediatric Hematology.* 2nd ed. London: Churchill Livingstone; 1999:651–678

Chapter 69

Elbow Deformity With Motor Deficit

Presentation

An 8-year-old girl is brought to the emergency department (ED) for a left elbow deformity. She had fallen with her arm in an unknown position 6 weeks previously. She had been traveling out of the country, and as a result of lack of local medical resources, her care was limited to radiographic diagnosis, an elastic wrap around the left elbow, and a sling.

Three weeks later, she returned to the United States. Her parents brought her to a local hospital, where no radiograph was obtained. The patient had 1 week of physical therapy and was lost to follow-up. On her visit to the ED, she has minimal pain, but she is unable to extend her arm completely and is experiencing some weakness in her left hand.

A nontender bony prominence arises from the medial aspect of the left elbow. Both hands are warm and well perfused. There is a valgus deformity of the left elbow with 45 degrees of flexion contracture (Figure 69-1). She is unable to flex at the proximal and distal interphalangeal joints of the index finger (flexor digitorum profundus and superficialis) and at the thumb interphalangeal joint (flexor pollicis longus) (Figure 69-2). Sensation is intact in all sensory distributions. She is able to abduct fingers and oppose the thumb. Pulses and perfusion are normal.

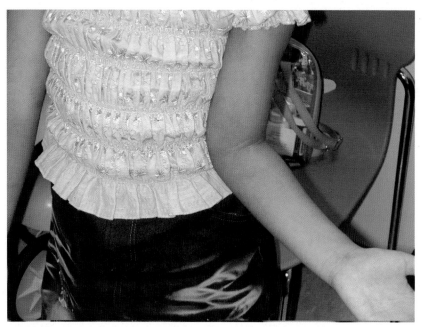

Figure 69-1

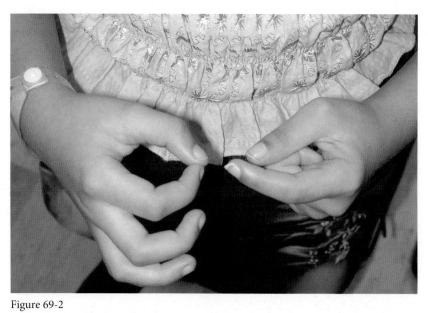

Figure 69-2

Discussion

Evaluation

You obtain the original x-ray films of the left elbow taken at the time of injury. They reveal a type 3 supracondylar fracture (Figure 69-3). This fracture is approximately 6 weeks old. The limb has not been placed in a cast, nor has surgical repair been offered. Now, the patient has a persistent deformity indicating bony malunion. Furthermore, weakness of the flexor digitorum profundus and superficialis muscles of the index finger and of the flexor pollicis longus provides evidence of neurologic deficit involving the anterior interosseous nerve.

Repeat films reveal an obvious deformity at the left humerus and a prominent callus over the fracture site (Figure 69-4).

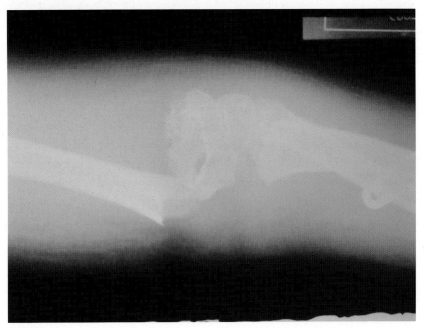

Figure 69-3

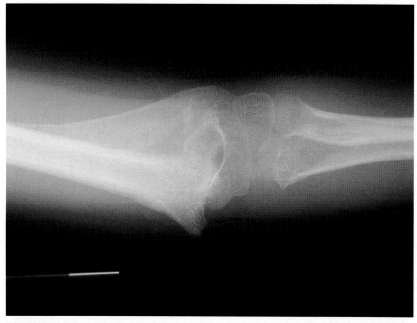

Figure 69-4

Treatment

Ordinary treatment of a displaced supracondylar humeral fracture includes timely operative reduction and fixation. Splint immobilization until the time of operative repair is standard. Because your patient's deformity is now stable, the orthopedic service recommends outpatient physical exercises and follow-up.

During follow-up, the patient has no complaints and she shows great improvement. She has a much better range of motion, and the affected hand has resumed normal function. Other than a residual valgus deformity, which produces a slight excess in carrying angle at the left elbow, the motor and sensory examinations are normal. Osteotomy would be required for correction. However, because range and function have returned, the family declines to pursue surgical correction because the residual deformity is purely cosmetic.

Keep in Mind

Supracondylar fractures are the most common elbow fractures in children, and prompt emergency stabilization and orthopedic care result in good outcomes. However, this injury has several notorious complications, including malunion, neurovascular injury, and compartment syndrome. Cubitus valgus, which occurred in this case, is much less common than cubitus varus (the so-called gunstock deformity). Although the persistent deformity is often considered cosmetic, it may predispose the patient to subsequent fracture.

For all but the most simple supracondylar fractures, operative reduction and fixation are recommended because the thinness of bone between olecranon and coronoid fossae leads to difficulty in maintaining reduction. Any of the nerves may be injured (up to 10%–15% of cases), and injury to the anterior interosseous nerve may be underrecognized as a result of the lack of concurrent sensory deficit. Detection of nerve injury may be difficult in younger and distressed patients, and it is wise to advise families that close orthopedic follow-up may be required to discover and treat these complications. Unexpectedly severe pain that persists after immobilization and analgesics, tense forearm compartments, and pain on passive extension of the fingers should alert the clinician to the possibility of compartment syndrome, even if distal pulses and capillary refill are normal.

Recommended Reading

Pring M, Rang M, Wenger D. Elbow—distal humerus. In: Wenger DR, Pring ME, eds. *Rang's Children's Fractures.* 3rd ed. Philadelphia, PA: Lippincott Williams & Wilkins; 2005:95–118

Upper extremity injuries. In: Herring JA, ed. *Tachdjian's Pediatric Orthopaedics.* 4th ed. Philadelphia, PA: Saunders Elsevier; 2008:2423–2572

Chapter 70

Limb Pain, Fever, and Anemia

Presentation

A 3-year-old boy arrives at the emergency department (ED) with a 3-week history of morning limb pain and a limp that persists through the rest of the day. The pain began in the right leg and migrated to the left. He cries when his parents pick him up or move his leg. There is no history of trauma and no limb swelling, rash, or bruising is present. His parents report that he has experienced intermittent unmeasured high temperatures for 3 weeks. Radiographs obtained by his primary care physician were normal, according to the parents' recollection. Ibuprofen provides some relief. A mild respiratory illness resolved 5 to 6 weeks previously without treatment. There is no family history of rheumatologic disorders or malignancy.

He is mildly febrile (temperature 38.3°C) and tachycardic (156 beats/min), but he appears well and is well perfused. His lungs are clear and other than tachycardia, the cardiovascular examination reveals nothing abnormal. His abdomen is soft with no hepatosplenomegaly or masses. He cries when you internally rotate his left hip and when you palpate his thighs, but no spine tenderness is evident. He limps slightly, keeping weight off his left leg. He has no rash, bruising, or adenopathy.

Discussion

Differential Diagnosis
- Septic arthritis
- Osteomyelitis
- Myositis
- Bacterial infection
- Transient synovitis
- Juvenile rheumatoid arthritis
- Malignancy

Evaluation
Screening studies reveal the following: white blood cells 9,000/μL (60% neutrophils, 5% band forms, and 23% lymphocytes), hemoglobin 9.2 g/dL, platelets 464,000/μL, erythrocyte sedimentation rate (ESR) greater than 140 mm/h, lactate dehydrogenase (LDH) 947 U/L (upper limit of normal range 950 U/L), creatine kinase 60 U/L (upper limit of normal range 91 U/L), and C-reactive protein (CRP) 4.6 mg/dL. Plain radiographs of the pelvis and left femur are normal (Figure 70-1). An orthopedic consultant arranges for admission, after which the patient remains afebrile without antibiotic therapy. Cultures of blood and left hip femoral neck aspirates yield no bacterial growth. A tuberculin skin test is negative. Results of tests for antinuclear antibodies, antistreptolysin antibodies, and complement levels are normal or negative. Despite an increase in CRP to 6.0 mg/dL, his pain improves rapidly when he is provided with naproxen, and he continues this medication as an outpatient for presumed transient synovitis or reactive arthritis.

Two months after his original visit, the patient returns to the ED with a headache, irritability, stiff neck, and fever to 38.3°C for 1 day. His parents report that he has decreased his oral intake but no respiratory symptoms, vomiting, or rash are evident. Between his 2 ED visits, he had visited his doctor to seek treatment for presumed constipation. A complete blood count at that time revealed a normocytic anemia (hemoglobin 8 gm/dL, mean corpuscular volume 81 fL) and prompted a course of iron therapy. His previous joint symptoms have not recurred. He is mildly febrile

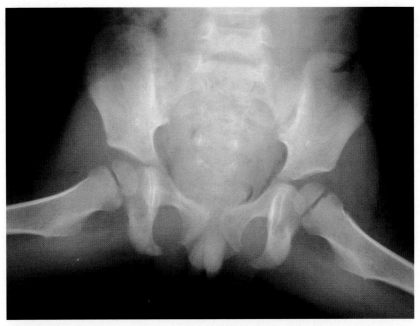

Figure 70-1

(38.4°C), tachycardic (120 beats/min), and very pale, but he appears well perfused. He has no cervical masses or adenopathy, but he will not flex or extend his neck. His abdomen is nontender with no distension or masses. His gait and extremity examination are normal.

On this ED visit, the differential diagnosis for the acute symptoms includes retropharyngeal abscess and meningitis. However, the previous symptoms and the anemia with marked pallor prompt you to reexamine the differential considerations of the first ED visit and admission. Laboratory findings include hemoglobin 5.6 gm/dL, normal white blood cell and platelet counts, CRP 8.2 mg/dL, ESR greater than 140 mm/h, and LDH 1,248 U/L. The reticulocyte count is 3.8%. Examination of cerebrospinal fluid is normal. A chest radiograph is normal, and a lateral soft tissue neck radiograph reveals no prevertebral soft tissue swelling.

You admit him to the general pediatric service and request consultation with specialists in rheumatology and oncology. After admission, he receives a transfusion, which improves his hemoglobin from 4.7 to 9.5 g/dL. Analysis of bone marrow biopsy samples reveals tumor cells suspicious for neuroblastoma. Computed tomography imaging reveals a left adrenal mass (Figure 70-2) and bony lesions of the skull. Skeletal scintigraphy reveals abnormal uptake in the right ilium, the left proximal femur, both distal femora, and the right clavicle (figures 70-3 and 70-4). Excisional biopsy of a retroperitoneal lymph node is performed, and analysis of the sample confirms the presence of metastatic neuroblastoma with unfavorable histology. Staging studies are consistent with metastatic neuroblastoma, with involvement of the abdominal-pelvic nodes, bone, and bone marrow. The boy undergoes chemotherapy, surgical excision of the residual tumor mass, and ultimately autologous peripheral blood stem cell transplantation 6 months after diagnosis.

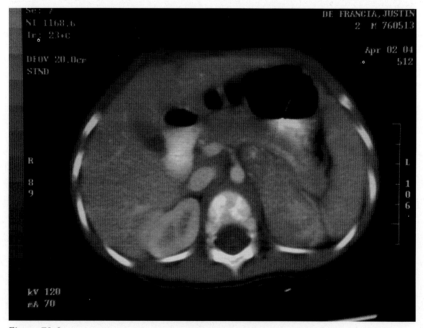

Figure 70-2

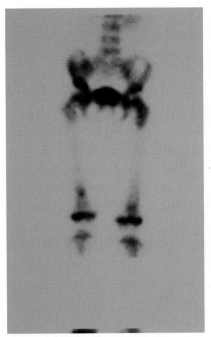
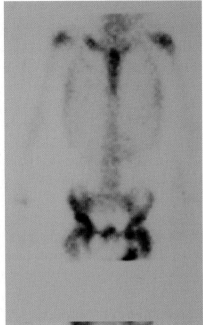

Figure 70-3   Figure 70-4

Keep in Mind

The presentation of neuroblastoma varies greatly with the location and size of the primary tumor as well as the degree of regional extension and metastatic spread. Abdominal primary tumors, especially those arising from the adrenal glands, are most common, but neuroblastomas may arise anywhere along the sympathetic chain. Compression by a tumor may cause venous obstruction including superior vena cava syndrome, Horner syndrome, spinal cord and nerve root deficits, and interference with bowel, bladder, and respiratory function. Metastatic disease is most common in bone, bone marrow, liver, and skin and may manifest with proptosis, periorbital ecchymosis, bone pain, marrow failure, failure to thrive and other systemic symptoms, and fever. Paraneoplastic phenomena include opsoclonus-myoclonus syndrome and intractable diarrhea.

Multiple ED or clinic visits suggest the need for more detailed investigation and possibly hospital admission. Similarly, abnormal laboratory results in a well-appearing patient warrant vigilant observation if the diagnosis and treatment plan are not immediately apparent.

Transient synovitis, a postinfectious reactive inflammation of the hip, is the most common cause of nontraumatic limp and limb pain in early childhood, and this provisional diagnosis may be appropriate for the limping child with no other physical findings when initial studies are normal. However, other categories of disease with important implications for treatment must be considered including infectious (eg, osteomyelitis, septic arthritis), neoplastic (eg, leukemia, neuroblastoma), rheumatologic (eg, juvenile idiopathic arthritis), and degenerative (eg, Legg-Calvé-Perthes disease) conditions. Typically, white blood cell count, ESR, and CRP are less elevated in transient synovitis than in bone and joint infections, and the condition improves rapidly and spontaneously, with the majority resolved by 2 weeks. In a small minority of patients, hip arthrocentesis is necessary to exclude septic arthritis with confidence.

Recommended Reading

Brodeur GM, Maris JM. Neuroblastoma. In: Pizzo PA, Poplack DG. *Principles and Practice of Pediatric Oncology.* 5th ed. Philadelphia, PA: Lippincott Williams & Wilkins; 2006:933–970

Kost S. Limp. In: Fleisher GR, Ludwig S, Henretig FM, Ruddy RM, Silverman BK, eds. *Textbook of Pediatric Emergency Medicine.* 5th ed. Philadelphia, PA: Lippincott Williams & Wilkins; 2006:415–420

Tunnessen WW, Roberts KB. Fever of undetermined origin. In: *Signs and Symptoms in Pediatrics.* 3rd ed. Philadelphia, PA: Lippincott Williams & Wilkins; 1999:3–7

Chapter 71

Thigh Pain and Weakness

Presentation

A 15-year-old girl presents with fever, body aches, and weakness. She had been well until yesterday, when she was noted to have a temperature of 38.5°C and complained of body aches. She was treated with acetaminophen, which resulted in improvement. Today, she vomited twice and had 2 episodes of diarrhea. Her body aches continued, with more pain in her left thigh. Her temperature was 39°C. She felt weak when she walking around, so she chose to lie down for most of the morning. Her mother noticed that she appeared to be slightly red, as if she had a sunburn, although she had not been out in the sun for at least 5 days. Her mother brought her to her primary care physician, who noticed that she felt faint when standing. He referred her to the emergency department for further evaluation.

Her oral intake has been poor and urine output is decreased. Her last menstrual period was 3 weeks ago. She denies that she is sexually active.

Past medical history is negative.

Your examination reveals the following vital signs: oral temperature 38.4°C, pulse 135 beats/min, respiration 30 breaths/min, blood pressure 85/55 mm Hg, and oxygen saturation 99% in room air. She is subdued and cooperative, in no distress. She is able to converse. Her eyes are not sunken. Her conjunctivae are clear. Tympanic membranes are normal and her oral mucosa is moist. Her pharynx is normal. Her neck is supple, without adenopathy. Heart examination reveals tachycardia with a grade 1/6 systolic murmur, but no gallop. Her lungs are clear. Her abdomen is soft and nontender. She has some mild tenderness in her left proximal thigh. Her hips have full range of motion with mild discomfort on the left. She complains of body aches in her back, neck, and upper arms; however, there is no tenderness when these areas are examined. She has a slight erythroderma that resembles a mild sunburn. Her skin is smooth without any sandpaper character. Her capillary refill time is roughly 2 seconds. When asked to stand up, she feels light-headed and asks to lie down again.

Discussion

Differential Diagnosis
- Staphylococcal toxic shock syndrome (TSS)
- Osteomyelitis
- Septic arthritis
- Viral syndrome

Evaluation
Orthostatic pulse and blood pressure measurements show mild orthostatic hypotension and tachycardia.

You order laboratory studies with the following findings: white blood cells 16,800/μL, 51% segmented neutrophils, 33% bands, 11% lymphocytes, 5% monocytes, hemoglobin 12 g/dL, hematocrit 36%, platelet count 180,000/μL, sodium 138 mmol/L, potassium 4.0 mmol/L, chloride 108 mmol/L, bicarbonate 12 mmol/L, blood urea nitrogen 20 mg/dL, creatinine 0.6 mg/dL, aspartate aminotransferase 30 U/L, alanine aminotransferase 40 U/L, and erythrocyte sedimentation rate 60 mm/h. A blood culture is pending.

Treatment
The patient is treated with an intravenous (IV) normal saline fluid bolus followed by a normal saline infusion and a dopamine infusion. She is given IV clindamycin and vancomycin. Her blood pressure and perfusion improve. Her light-headedness improves. A magnetic resonance imaging scan identifies an early osteomyelitis of her proximal left femur. An aspirate of the affected femur region and her blood culture both grow *Staphylococcus aureus.*

She is admitted to the intensive care unit. During hospitalization, she continues to improve, and her skin undergoes mild desquamation, most pronounced in her palms and soles approximately 1 week later.

Although her signs and symptoms of early shock could be because of septic shock, you diagnose her with TSS because of the erythroderma. *S aureus* can cause septic shock as well, but most patients with early staphylococcal osteomyelitis have not progressed to septic shock.

Keep in Mind

Staphylococcal TSS was first described in 1978. Before this, TSS was not an established diagnosis, and poor outcomes were attributed to other erythroderma conditions that were more typically benign.

Most initial cases of staphylococcal TSS were associated with tampon use. An epidemic of TSS was associated with the introduction of superabsorbent tampons. These have since been removed from the market, resulting in a marked decline in TSS.

Staphylococci are known to cause other toxin-related diseases, such as staphylococcal scalded skin syndrome, bullous impetigo, and staphylococcal food poisoning.

The findings in staphylococcal TSS include fever, rash (a diffuse erythroderma followed by desquamation, as seen in this patient), hypotension, tachycardia, vomiting, diarrhea, myalgias, mucous membrane hyperemia, azotemia, high liver enzyme values, thrombocytopenia, and other signs and symptoms of shock. Measles, Kawasaki disease, Rocky Mountain spotted fever, and leptospirosis can be included in the differential diagnosis, depending on the specific pattern of signs and symptoms. The clinical case definition of TSS is outlined in Table 71-1.

The focus of the staphylococcal infection may appear surprisingly benign, such as sinusitis, impetigo, or paronychia. The toxin interferes with the release of inflammatory mediators, so signs of inflammation may be absent.

Early recognition of shock and aggressive treatment to prevent the stage of shock from advancing improves outcome. This applies to staphylococcal TSS. These patients generally require intensive care unit monitoring and treatment with inotrope infusions.

Table 71-1. *Staphylococcus aureus* **Toxic Shock Syndrome: Clinical Case Definition[a]**

Clinical Findings
• Fever: temperature 38.9°C (102.0°F) or greater
• Rash: diffuse macular erythroderma
• Desquamation: 1–2 wk after onset, particularly on palms, soles, fingers, and toes
• Hypotension: systolic pressure 90 mm Hg or less for adults; lower than fifth percentile for age for children younger than 16 years of age; orthostatic drop in diastolic pressure of 15 mm Hg or greater from lying to sitting; orthostatic syncope or orthostatic dizziness
• Multisystem organ involvement: 3 or more of the following: – Gastrointestinal: vomiting or diarrhea at onset of illness   – Muscular: severe myalgia or creatinine phosphokinase concentration greater than twice the upper limit of normal   – Mucous membrane: vaginal, oropharyngeal, or conjunctival hyperemia   – Renal: serum urea nitrogen or serum creatinine concentration greater than twice the upper limit of normal or urinary sediment with 5 white blood cells/high-power field or greater in the absence of urinary tract infection   – Hepatic: total bilirubin, aspartate transaminase, or alanine transaminase concentration greater than twice the upper limit of normal   – Hematologic: platelet count 100 000/mm 3 or less   – Central nervous system: disorientation or alterations in consciousness without focal neurologic signs when fever and hypotension are absent

Laboratory Criteria
• *Negative* results on the following tests, if obtained: – Blood, throat, or cerebrospinal fluid cultures; blood culture may be positive for *S aureus*   – Serologic tests for Rocky Mountain spotted fever, leptospirosis, or measles

Case Classification
• **Probable:** a case that meets the laboratory criteria and in which 4 of 5 clinical findings are present
• **Confirmed:** a case that meets laboratory criteria and all 5 of the clinical findings, including desquamation, unless the patient dies before desquamation occurs.

[a] Adapted from Wharton M, Chorba TL, Vogt RL, Morse DL, Buehler JW. Case definitions for public health surveillance. *MMWR Recomm Rep.* 1990;39(RR-13):1–43

Recommended Reading

Vincent JM. Staphylococcal and streptococcal toxic shock syndromes.
In: Yamamoto LG, Inaba AS, Okamoto JK, Patronis ME, Yamashiroya
VK, eds. *Case Based Pediatrics for Medical Students and Residents.*
Honolulu, HI: University of Hawaii; 2004:199–203. Available at: http://
www.hawaii.edu/medicine/pediatrics/pedtext. Accessed December 31,
2008

Part 8

Genital/Rectal Conditions

Chapter 72

Genital Pain

Presentation

An 8-year-old girl has experienced genital pain of several hours' duration. One of the hairs from her head had fallen into her underwear and wrapped around the distal clitoris and adjacent labia minora. Her mother unsuccessfully attempted to remove the hair. Over the ensuing hours, the girl experienced progressive swelling and discoloration of the entrapped portion, and she reports pain with urination.

Genital examination reveals edema and violet-colored discoloration of the distal clitoris. She complains of pain with palpation. Close inspection reveals a hair tourniquet around the clitoris, with fibers embedded in the skin (Figure 72-1).

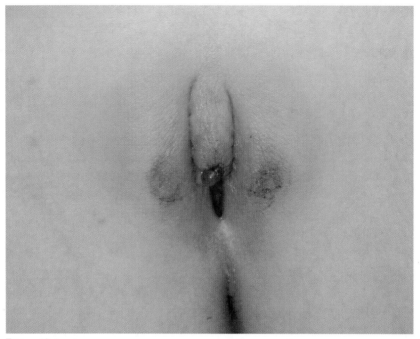

Figure 72-1

Discussion

Evaluation

On examination, the diagnosis is not in question. However, clinicians should make an effort to exclude inflicted causes of a genital injury or foreign body.

Treatment

Your examination suggests that removal by elevation and division of the constricting fibers is feasible. Despite a surprising degree of patient cooperation, she continues to experience discomfort and pain that interferes with successful removal. A topical application of 4% liposomal lidocaine for 30 minutes permits painless manipulation. The embedded hairs are elevated from the skin with forceps and divided with a scalpel blade. Normal perfusion returns, and swelling and pain quickly resolve (Figure 72-2).

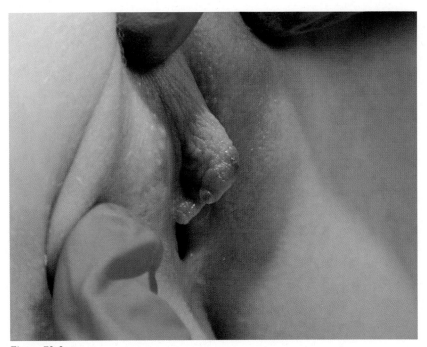

Figure 72-2

Keep in Mind

Although this hair tourniquet occurred on the genitalia of a school-aged child, most occur on the toes of small infants. In the preverbal child, a digit or genital hair tourniquet may be the unsuspected cause of persistent crying. A gentle, unhurried approach combined with topical anesthetic often allows the clinician to avoid deep sedation or general anesthesia in treating soft tissue emergencies. Application of a depilatory may be useful for some hair tourniquets.

A penile hair tourniquet is removed in a similar fashion. The hairs may be isolated and divided more easily because of the larger diameter of the ensnared organ. Skin adjacent to the fibers may be depressed, allowing relatively painless and atraumatic use of scissors or scalpel.

Recommended Reading

Loiselle JM, Cronan KM. Hair tourniquet removal. In: King C, Henretig FM, King BR, Loiselle JM, Ruddy RM, Wiley JF, eds. *Textbook of Pediatric Emergency Procedures.* 2nd ed. Philadelphia, PA: Lippincott Williams & Wilkins; 2008:1065–1069

Chapter 73

Penile Swelling

Presentation

A 13-year-old boy is referred to the emergency department (ED) by an outlying clinic for penile swelling of 4 days' duration. The penile swelling started after masturbation 4 days before. He did not tell his parents about it until 2 days later, when the swelling worsened and it became very painful. He was assessed in a clinic that prescribed cephalexin and topical nystatin powder. It did not improve, so he was assessed again yesterday and was given a single dose of intramuscular dexamethasone. The swelling and pain continued to worsen and he returned to the clinic, at which point he was referred to the ED. There is no history of fever, vomiting, diarrhea, cold symptoms, or dysuria. He is uncircumcised.

Past medical history is negative.

Your examination reveals the following vital signs: oral temperature 37.0°C, pulse 94 beats/min, respiration 18 breaths/min, and blood pressure 120/65 mm Hg. He is alert and cooperative. He denies current pain. Heart, lung, and abdominal examinations are negative. He has no inguinal hernias. His scrotum is normal. He penis is swollen and edematous. The perfusion and color of the glans are good (Figure 73-1). The white powder is nystatin powder.

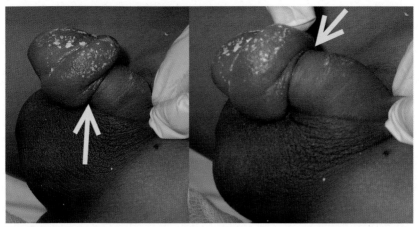

Figure 73-1

Discussion

Differential Diagnosis
• Paraphimosis

Evaluation
The glans is slightly swollen but its perfusion is good. The patient has been able to urinate. Thus, the initial examiners thought that this was not a case of paraphimosis because there was no obvious venous engorgement. However, in this case, the paraphimosis ring is not tight enough to cause venous obstruction. Additionally, the constricting ring is hidden under the edematous ring of tissue proximal to the glans. Figure 73-1 shows the constricting ring that can be viewed once this edematous tissue is retracted distally. The key diagnostic point is that if the patient is uncircumcised, where is the foreskin? If it is not visible, paraphimosis should be suspected. In Figure 73-1, the foreskin is irreversibly retracted and constricting the penile shaft, which is the hallmark of paraphimosis.

Treatment
A urologist is consulted. A penile block is applied. The paraphimosis is reduced by squeezing the edema from the distal penis after the penile block took effect.

Keep in Mind

Paraphimosis is defined as a condition in which the distal foreskin is retracted proximal to the glans, resulting in constriction of the penis. The white arrows in Figure 73-1 show the constricting band of tissue proximal to the swollen ring of tissue.

Phimosis refers to the condition in which the foreskin cannot be fully retracted to expose the glans. This is normal in the newborn. In the following years, the retractability of the foreskin increases until it can be retracted fully.

Pathologic phimosis refers to a condition in which the foreskin cannot be retracted as a result of pathologic factors such as cellulitis with scarring of the foreskin. Physiologic phimosis is normal in newborns and gradually resolves.

Paraphimosis is an emergent condition in which the foreskin is retracted proximal to the glans and cannot be returned to its normal position. Common causes include forceful retraction of the foreskin (sometimes done during urethral catheterization for urine collection), normal hygiene, and sexual stimulation. If the retracted foreskin is not returned to its normal position, vascular congestion results in swelling and constriction of the penile shaft. At this point, it may be difficult or impossible for the foreskin to be returned to its normal position. Topical anesthetic cream followed by pressure on the glans and swollen prepuce to reduce edema can often permit reduction of the paraphimosis. More difficult reductions can be accomplished under deep sedation, general anesthesia, or an extensive penile block. Although paraphimosis can be reduced by the primary care or emergency physician in many instances, emergency consultation with a urologist or pediatric surgeon is often necessary for difficult reductions.

The key is to identify a paraphimosis at its early stage. The foreskin should be clearly visible in the uncircumcised penis. If it is not visible or if it cannot be returned to its normal position over the glans, paraphimosis is likely.

Recommended Reading

Snyder HM. Urologic emergencies. In: Fleisher GR, Ludwig S, Henretig FM, Ruddy RM, Silverman BK, eds. *Textbook of Pediatric Emergency Medicine*. 5th ed. Philadelphia, PA: Lippincott Williams & Wilkins; 2006:1679–1687

Chapter 74

Anal Mass

Presentation

Earlier today, a 3-year-old boy sought care at his primary care physician's office for an anal mass. He had a history of hard stools and had several previous instances of a red doughnut of tissue protruding from his anus while straining to stool, but by the time they were seen by his doctor, the red doughnut had gone back into his anus. His mother thought that it was a large hemorrhoid, but his primary care physician advised her that it was probably a prolapsing rectum. Today was the first time that he arrived in the office with the rectum still prolapsed. As usual, it occurred while he was straining to stool. The boy's mother reported that her son had no history of vomiting, fever, pain, or coughing. He was eating well. His primary care physician attempted to reduce the rectal prolapse, but because the boy was crying during the reduction attempt, it was not successful. His primary care physician referred him to the emergency department (ED) for another reduction attempt.

Past medical history is negative except for hard stools and recurrent rectal prolapse by history.

Your examination reveals the following vital signs: axillary temperature 37.4°C, pulse 110 beats/min, respiration 30 breaths/min, blood pressure 90/60 mm Hg, and oxygen saturation 99% in room air. He is fairly cooperative and not irritable. Examination of head, eyes, ears, nose, and throat reveals nothing abnormal. Heart and lungs are normal. His abdomen is soft and nontender. He has no inguinal hernias. His external genitalia are normal. A complete rectal prolapse is visible (Figure 74-1). The tissue is pink/red rather than pale/blue.

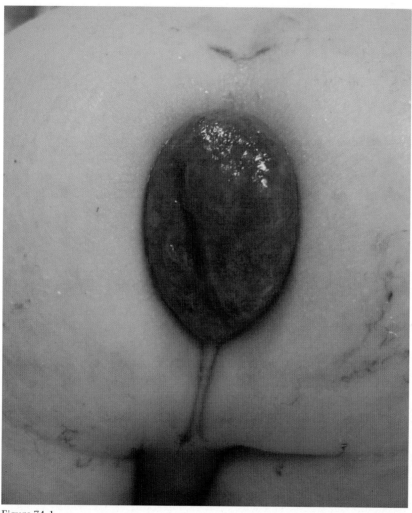

Figure 74-1

Discussion

Differential Diagnosis
- Rectal prolapse
- Intussusception

Evaluation

The patient is assessed for sedation options. You discuss sedation and analgesia options with his mother. His primary care physician has already tried to reduce the prolapsed rectum and was unsuccessful, so you conclude that it is likely that the reduction will be difficult. Sedation or analgesia will probably facilitate the reduction. Some of your options include an oral narcotic analgesic, a parenteral narcotic analgesic, or other nonnarcotic sedative or analgesic options such as ketamine or propofol. The best option is not immediately obvious. An oral narcotic analgesic such as acetaminophen with oxycodone might be effective. Deep sedation with propofol is more likely to completely sedate the patient, but this option might deliver more sedation than the patient needs.

Treatment

After a discussion of sedation and analgesic options with the patient's mother, together you decide on intravenous (IV) morphine. When the IV morphine is provided, the patient is completely awake but more cooperative. He is placed in a prone position and his knees are brought forward to his chest, buttocks facing upward. Broad pressure is applied to the prolapsed rectum and it is fairly easily reduced. The patient does not complain of any pain and cooperates with the procedure despite being completely awake. He tolerates the procedure well. After 10 minutes, he is drinking juice and continues to be alert and active, and the prolapse has not recurred. He is discharged from the ED with a stool-softening regimen.

Keep in Mind

Rectal prolapse is fairly uncommon. Mucosal bleeding is common. Causes include constipation, diarrhea, and cystic fibrosis. Most patients do not require surgical repair. Recurrences are common.

Conditions that mimic rectal prolapse include intussusception (the intussusceptum has intussuscepted from the cecum all the way to anus). A urethral prolapse can mimic a rectal prolapse in girls, except that the prolapse clearly comes from the vagina and not the anus.

Reduction is facilitated with sedation or analgesia. Crying makes reduction difficult. Reduction can generally be accomplished with a gentle approach and broad-based pressure applied to the entire prolapse.

Another technique for reduction includes wrapping a gloved index finger with toilet tissue. When this finger is inserted into the rectum, the tissue pulls the prolapsed rectal tissue inward. The toilet tissue can be left inside the rectum once reduction is achieved.

Recommended Reading

Chung SA. Minor lesions and injuries. In: Fleisher GR, Ludwig S, Henretig FM, Ruddy RM, Silverman BK, eds. *Textbook of Pediatric Emergency Medicine.* 5th ed. Philadelphia, PA: Lippincott Williams & Wilkins; 2006:1589–1604

Santamaria J. Office-based procedures. Section 5. Miscellaneous procedures. In: Gausche-Hill M, Fuchs S, Yamamoto L, eds. *APLS: The Pediatric Emergency Medicine Resource.* 4th rev ed. Sudbury, MA: Jones and Bartlett Publishers; 2007:662–672

Schwartz G. Reducing a rectal prolapse. In: King C, Henretig FM, eds. *Textbook of Pediatric Emergency Procedures.* 2nd ed. Philadelphia, PA: Lippincott Williams & Wilkins; 2008:859–862

Part 9

Pulmonary Presentations

Chapter 75

Is That a Tension Pneumothorax?

Presentation

A 2-week-old baby boy is brought to the emergency department with difficulty breathing today; he appears to be struggling to breathe. His parents think that he stops breathing sometimes and turns blue. When they stimulate him, he starts breathing again. He has no coughing, runny nose, fever, vomiting, or diarrhea.

Past medical history reveals that he was born at term, with a birth weight of 3.5 kg. No risk factors for sepsis are evident. His parents thought that his breathing pattern was abnormal, but because this is their first child, this concern was dismissed. The parents describe the abnormal breathing pattern as breathing fast, sometimes with his chest caving in deeply.

Your examination reveals the following vital signs: temperature 36.7°C, pulse 160 beats/min, respiration 60 breaths/min, blood pressure 100/70 mm Hg, and oxygen saturation 86% in room air. Oxygen is applied, and his oxygen saturation is now 100%. He is alert with obvious tachypnea and retractions. There are no signs of external trauma. His nose is clear and there is no nasal flaring. Suprasternal, intercostal, and subcostal retractions are present. Breath sounds are diminished throughout the chest, indicating poor aeration, but you do not hear any wheezing. His heart tones are distant and you do not hear a murmur. His abdominal contour is normal. His pulses are strong and regular. Overall perfusion is good.

Discussion

Differential Diagnosis
- Pneumonia
- Pneumothorax
- Chylothorax
- Pulmonary congenital anomaly
- Congenital heart disease
- Tracheomalacia
- Airway anomaly

Evaluation
You immediately order a chest radiograph, which reveals hyperlucency of the left chest with a substantial mediastinal/cardiac shift to the right (Figure 75-1). Your initial impression is that this is a tension pneumothorax, and you decide to attempt a needle thoracentesis. However, one of your colleagues questions this decision.

Treatment
Pending further evaluation, you continue the supplemental oxygen, relieving the child's hypoxia.

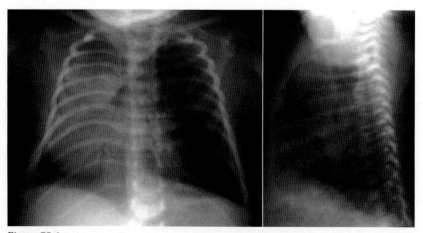

Figure 75-1

Your colleague points out that the usual cause of a tension pneumothorax is positive pressure ventilation (ventilator) or penetrating external trauma. Although it is possible to have a tension pneumothorax without these factors, it is uncommon. A tension pneumothorax generally results in sudden deterioration with severe hypoxia and hypotension that is refractory to all treatments except for relief of the tension by thoracentesis or tube thoracostomy. However, this particular patient's blood pressure is good, and his hypoxia is easily remedied by applying an oxygen mask. A true tension pneumothorax results in rapid deterioration such that the patient will generally die before a chest radiograph can confirm the presence of a tension pneumothorax. Thus, for this newborn, multiple factors are inconsistent with a tension pneumothorax.

You examine the chest radiograph more closely, but it is difficult to come to a conclusion. In actuality, this patient has a hyperexpanded lobe due to congenital lobar emphysema. In this condition, a lobar bronchial airway is floppy and a one-way valve phenomenon develops such that the lobe traps air. As the infant inhales more, more air is trapped in the lobe, and the lobe hyperexpands to compress the normal portions of the lung. The hyperexpanded left chest is a single hyperexpanded emphysematous left upper lobe. The remainder of the left lung is compressed and difficult to visualize on the chest radiograph. The hyperexpanded left upper lobe shifts the mediastinum to the right, partially compressing the right lung. Fortunately, the heart is not as easily compressed, permitting sufficient circulation. These phenomena are similar to what occurs in a tension pneumothorax, but not as severe.

A needle thoracentesis or tube thoracostomy will not help this condition because there is no air leak into the pleural space. Puncturing the emphysematous lobe will not deflate it. Definitive treatment requires surgical removal of the emphysematous lobe.

Recommended Reading

Kelly RE, Isaacman DJ. Thoracic emergencies. In: Fleisher GR, Ludwig S, Henretig FM, Ruddy RM, Silverman BK, eds. *Textbook of Pediatric Emergency Medicine.* 5th ed. Philadelphia, PA: Lippincott Williams & Wilkins; 2006:1631–1651

Rosen LM. Respiratory distress—that's a tension pneumothorax, isn't it? In: Yamamoto LG, Inaba AS, DiMauro R, eds. *Radiology Cases in Pediatric Emergency Medicine.* Vol 1, case 9. November 1994. Available at: http://www.hawaii.edu/medicine/pediatrics/pemxray/v1c09.html. Accessed December 31, 2008

Chapter 76

Difficulty Breathing and Fever

Presentation

A 3-week-old boy is brought to the emergency department (ED) by his mother because of difficulty breathing and fever (axillary temperature, 38.1°C). He has vomited twice today. He was well yesterday. He is slightly fussy with a mild cough and decreased appetite. His urine output is unchanged. There is no history of diarrhea. His parents administered an albuterol aerosol at home, but this treatment did not seem to help.

Past medical history is significant for a single episode of wheezing, treated with albuterol aerosols.

Examination reveals the following vital signs: rectal temperature 38.4°C, pulse 234 beats/min, respiration 55 breaths/min (while crying), blood pressure unobtainable, and oxygen saturation 99% in room air. He is alert and active, and in mild distress. He is not toxic and not excessively irritable. Anterior fontanelle is small and flat. His eyes are moist, not sunken. His oral mucosa is moist. His tympanic membranes are slightly red. His neck is supple. His heart is tachycardic with no obvious murmur. His lungs exhibit mild wheezing, few rales, good aeration, and slight retractions. His abdomen is soft and flat with active bowel sounds. His liver edge is difficult to identify. No inguinal hernias are present. His color and perfusion are good. Capillary refill is 1.5 to 2 seconds. He is moving all his extremities well and his muscle tone is good.

An electrocardiogram (ECG) is obtained (Figure 76-1).

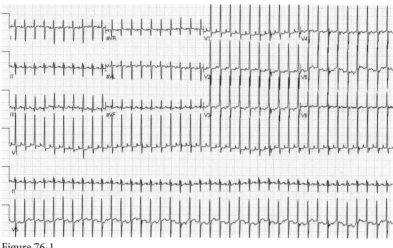

Figure 76-1

Discussion

Differential Diagnosis

- Wheezing
- Respiratory infection
- Pneumonia
- Bronchiolitis
- Congestive heart failure
- Paroxysmal supraventricular tachycardia (PSVT)
- Sinus tachycardia (ST)

Evaluation

You interpret the ECG as follows: the rate is 238 per minute. The axis is rightward, which is not unusual for a young infant. The QRS is narrow. There are smaller waves in-between the QRS complexes. These are more likely to be T waves and not P waves. These waves might actually be 2 fused waves, further confusing the issue.

Treatment

An albuterol aerosol is administered in the ED. The patient's clinical status remains roughly the same. A complete blood count, blood culture, and chemistry panel are obtained. A urinalysis and urine culture are obtained. A lumbar puncture is considered, but you and his parents decide to hold off on this for now. Intravenous (IV) antibiotics are provided. A major clinical issue is to determine whether the tachycardia is caused by an ST versus a PSVT.

This patient has many reasons to have an ST. He has a fever, he is exhibiting respiratory distress, and he has received 2 albuterol treatments.

Distinguishing ST from PSVT can be difficult. Table 76-1 lists some of the distinguishing criteria.

The patient's heart rate of 234 beats/min is compatible with a PSVT or a very fast ST. His high temperature, respiratory distress, and albuterol treatments could drive his heart rate up to 234 beats/min. If his heart rate increases substantially with crying, followed by a significant decline when his crying subsides, this would be more compatible with an ST. If his heart rate stays relatively unchanged with crying, PSVT is more likely.

Although the albuterol treatment will often increase the patient's heart rate, it might also reduce his degree of respiratory distress if he has a significant degree of bronchospasm. Administering an antipyretic will likely

Table 76-1. Criteria Distinguishing Sinus Tachycardia From Paroxysmal Supraventricular Tachycardia

Criterion	Sinus Tachycardia	Paroxysmal Supraventricular Tachycardia
Heart rate	<2 times heart rate for age	>2 times heart rate for age
Heart rate variability	Heart rate varies with stimuli and treatments.	Heart rate does not vary much with stimuli and treatments.
P wave	P waves are present.	P waves are absent.
History	Suggestive of sinus tachycardia (eg, fever, hypovolemia, beta agents)	History of paroxysmal supraventricular tachycardia
Response to vagal maneuver	Slow decline	If successful, sudden conversion
Response to adenosine	No response	Sudden conversion

reduce his temperature and his heart rate if this is an ST. Because his history does not suggest significant volume depletion, hypovolemia is not suspected. However, if hypovolemia is the cause of an ST, administering a fluid bolus should result in a gradual decline in the patient's heart rate as euvolemia is restored.

In this case, the patient's heart rate has remained fairly stable despite his temperature normalizing. Therefore, PSVT is suspected. His circulation is satisfactory at this time, so a vagal maneuver is indicated initially. Vagal maneuvers include ice to the face and scalp (the diving reflex), Valsalva, carotid massage, and eyeball pressure. The diving reflex results in the greatest degree of vagal simulation compared with the other vagal maneuvers. The diving reflex is the favored vagal maneuver for children. This is accomplished by applying a bag of slushy ice to the face and scalp. If this results in conversion to a sinus rhythm, the ECG typically shows a brief period of asystole followed by a sinus rhythm. In this case, a vagal maneuver is attempted without success. The tachycardia persists.

The next indicated therapeutic intervention is IV adenosine. The effect of adenosine is optimized by very rapid bolus. This is facilitated by a rapid push-and-flush technique. A common method of accomplishing this is to use a 2-syringe and stopcock setup (Figure 76-2). The adenosine syringe is injected rapidly; the stopcock-off lever is then rapidly moved from the position to occlude the saline (3-o'clock position in the figure), to the position to occlude the adenosine (12-o'clock position in the figure); then the saline syringe is injected rapidly to flush in the adenosine. This sequence of events should be conducted as rapidly as possible to create a very rapid bolus of adenosine.

This process can also be facilitated by elevating the extremity with the IV. This permits the adenosine bolus to flow intravenously downhill into the body and central circulation rather than flowing level or uphill into the body.

Some clinicians have commented that the setup shown in Figure 76-3 results in a faster bolus injection of adenosine. Large bore needles are attached via Luer lock to an adenosine syringe and a saline flush syringe.

Both needles are inserted into a rubber injection port as close to the IV site as possible. To facilitate a rapid bolus of adenosine, the administrator must hold the plunger of the saline syringe (to prevent the adenosine from entering the saline syringe) while the adenosine syringe is rapidly pushed, followed immediately by a rapid push of the saline syringe while holding the adenosine syringe plunger. Note that the blue tubing clip (figures 76-3 and 76-4) must also close the IV infusion line so that the adenosine bolus proceeds forward toward the patient's vein, rather than flowing backward into the IV fluid bag.

An adenosine bolus is administered that results in a brief asystolic pause, followed by a sustained sinus rhythm of 105 beats/min. Postconversion ECGs will sometimes reveal underlying causes of PSVT such as Wolff-Parkinson-White syndrome, characterized by a short P–R interval and a delta wave.

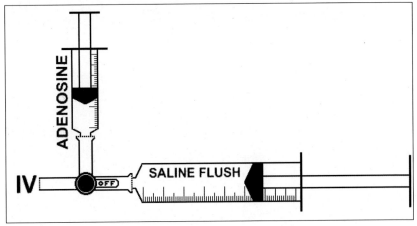

Figure 76-2

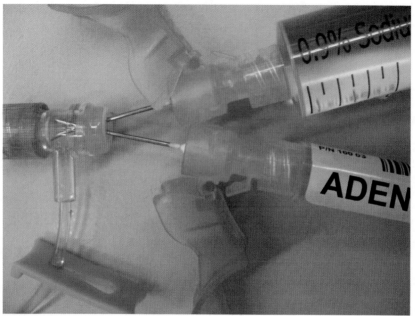

Figure 76-3

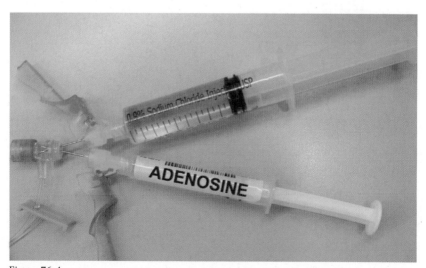

Figure 76-4

Keep in Mind

Consultation with a cardiologist can help to determine whether electro-physiological interventions might be necessary. Drug prophylaxis with propranolol or digoxin is commonly recommended. Propranolol is a beta-receptor antagonist, so it is contraindicated in patients with asthma. Digoxin is potentially contraindicated in some patients with Wolff-Parkinson-White syndrome.

Recommended Reading

Berk WA, Shea MJ, Crevey BJ. Bradycardic responses to vagally mediated bedside maneuvers in healthy volunteers. *Am J Med*. 1991;90:725–729

Fitzmaurice L, Gerardi MJ. Cardiovascular system. In: Gausche-Hill M, Fuchs S, Yamamoto L, eds. *APLS: The Pediatric Emergency Medicine Resource*. 4th rev ed. Sudbury, MA: Jones and Bartlett Publishers; 2007:106–145

Chapter 77

Stridor for 2 Weeks

Presentation

An 11-month-old girl arrives in the emergency department with a 2-week history of noisy respirations with no fever. Her mother reports that rhinorrhea has been present during this time, and the sounds have been worsening recently. She has not vomited and has been eating without difficulty. She has been previously healthy with no history of respiratory problems, hemangiomas, or other soft tissue tumors. Family history is negative for childhood cardiac or pulmonary disease. She is afebrile, alert, vigorous, and well perfused with room air oxyhemoglobin saturations of 97%. You note mild to moderate low-pitched biphasic stridor during rapid or deep respiration. However, no stridor occurs when she is resting quietly or asleep. Skin examination reveals no hemangiomas.

Discussion

Differential Diagnosis
- Croup
- Epiglottitis
- Tracheitis
- Functional and structural airway anomalies such as laryngomalacia or vocal cord paralysis
- Acquired airway lesions such as papilloma or hemangioma
- Foreign body
- Airway trauma
- Retropharyngeal abscess
- Psychogenic disorder (in older children and adolescents)
- Vascular ring

Evaluation
Soft tissue neck radiographs reveal no foreign body or soft tissue abnormalities. Chest radiographs reveal no foreign body. However, a subtle indentation appears on the right side of the midthoracic trachea, and it persists on repeat films (Figure 77-1). Tracheal compression raises the possibility of a vascular ring. Subsequent computed tomography (CT) imaging reveals a right-sided aortic arch (Figure 77-2) that causes marked compression of the trachea (Figure 77-3). Echocardiography reveals a double aortic arch

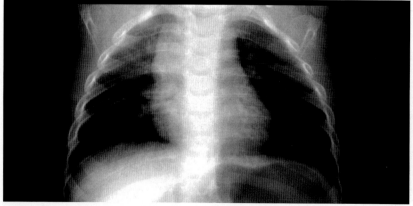

Figure 77-1

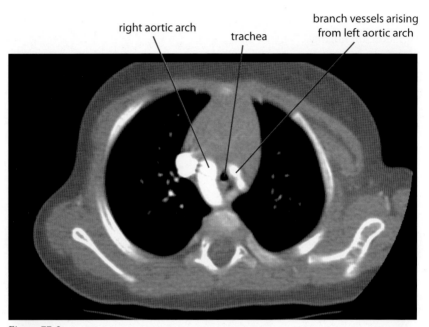

Figure 77-2

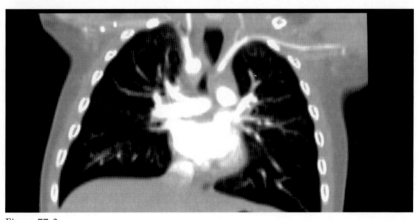

Figure 77-3

and normal coronary anatomy. The intracardiac anatomy and ventricular function are normal.

You diagnose the girl with a vascular ring.

Treatment
The patient undergoes repair of the vascular ring with division of an atretic left aortic arch and ligamentum arteriosum, and has an uneventful recovery.

Keep in Mind
Not all stridor represents croup when it is acute, nor tracheomalacia when it is long-standing.

Vascular rings may be complete (eg, double aortic arch, right arch with left ligamentum arteriosum) or incomplete (eg, anomalous innominate artery, aberrant right subclavian artery, anomalous right pulmonary artery). The vascular ring present in this patient—a double aortic arch with a dominant right arch—is the most common. Because the ring completely surrounds and compresses the trachea and esophagus, the absence of feeding difficulties or previous respiratory symptoms is unusual in this patient. However, age at onset and severity of symptoms vary with degree of compression by the ring, and some asymptomatic lesions are discovered incidentally.

Chest radiography may reveal tracheal compression as well as pneumonia or atelectasis. More definitive diagnostic studies include contrast esophagography and CT. Echocardiography will define the vascular anatomy and detect intracardiac defects in about a quarter of cases. Laryngoscopy and bronchoscopy are more useful in the evaluation of intrinsic anatomic and functional problems of the airway, but these techniques may demonstrate a pulsatile indentation caused by the ring.

Recommended Reading

Park MK. Vascular ring. In: *Pediatric Cardiology for Practitioners.* 5th ed. Philadelphia, PA: CV Mosby; 2008:303–308

Weinberg PM. Aortic arch anomalies. In: Allen HD, Shaddy RE, Driscoll DJ, Feltes TF, ed. *Moss and Adams' Heart Disease in Infants, Children, and Adolescents: Including the Fetus and Young Adult.* 7th ed. Philadelphia, PA: Lippincott Williams & Wilkins; 2008:730–760

Index